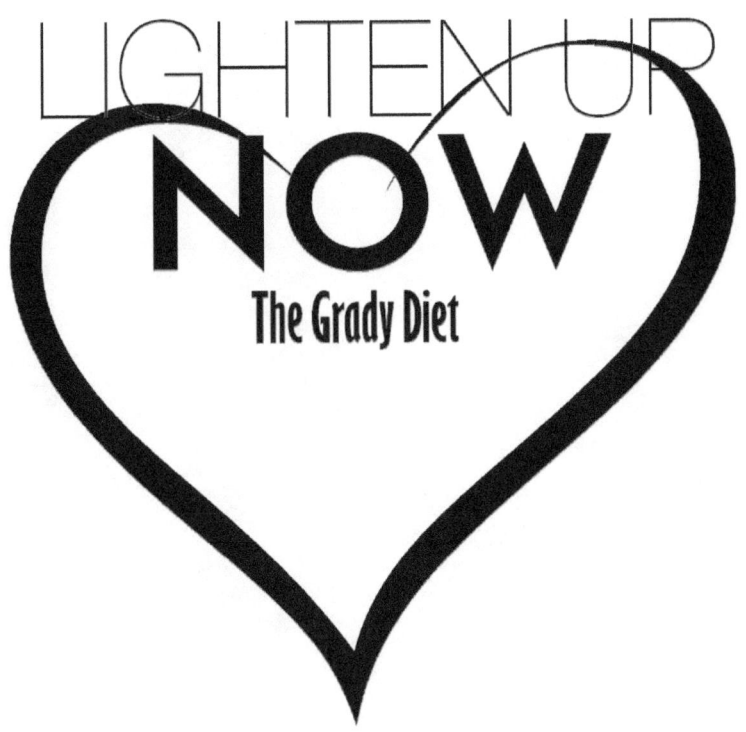

LIGHTEN UP

NOW

The Grady Diet

LIGHTEN UP NOW

The Grady Diet

A DIET TO LIGHTEN UP YOUR MIND & BODY

GRADY MILLER

GRADY MILLER BOOKS

LIGHTEN UP NOW: The Grady Diet

Copyright © 2013 by Grady Miller

AUTHOR'S PHOTO by Don Goodman
(**ship2me@gmail.com**)

COVER DESIGN by Vivek Rajan Vivek
(**vivek.rajan.vivek@gmail.com**)

"Malibu Grady" PHOTO by Jeffrey Davis
(**zepherzen3@hotmail.com**)

INTERIOR COVER DESIGN by Yevgen Kaminsky
(**yevgenkaminsky@gmail.com**)

Please contact the publisher at: **gradytrain@hotmail.com**

1236 1/8 N. Cahuenga Blvd.
Hollywood, CA 90038

To Mom

You bought all the diet books
that ever were. I'm giving
you this one, with love.

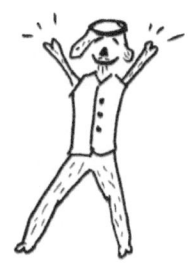

Contents

Foreword xiii

1 INTRODUCTION: *Love Yourself First* 15

2 AFTER: *From Fat to Emaciated in 30 Days* 27

3 BODY CHANGER: *Morning Exercise* 39

4 100 LAUGHS: *Making It, Faking It, Doing It* 43

5 THE SEVEN STEPS: *Sparky's Ladder* 53

6 BEFORE: *From Emaciated to Fat in 30 Days* 77

7 I'M NOT A VEGETARIAN: *And More Secrets* 83

8 GROWING YOUR OWN: *Hollywood Style* 89

9 BACKWARD: *The Grady Story* 95

10 THE GRADY KOOKBOOK 109

THANKS YOUS 135

ABOUT THE AUTHOR 136

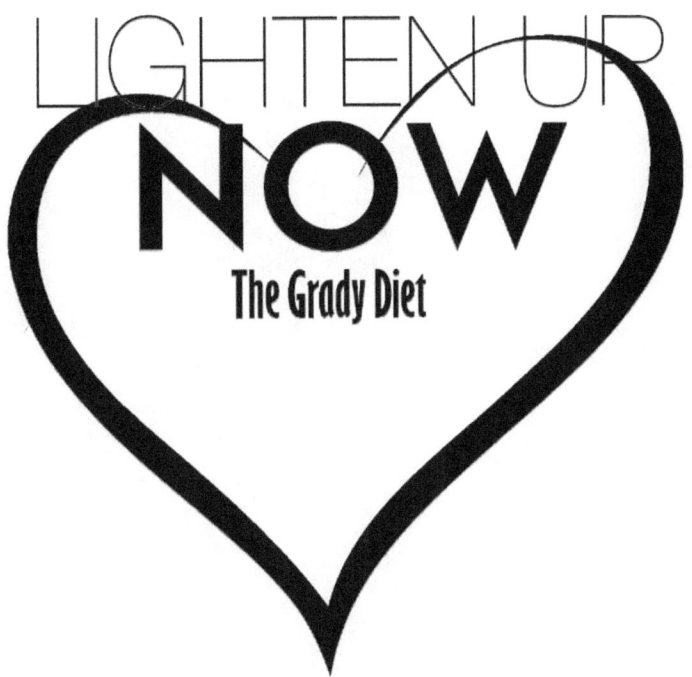

Foreword

Lighten Up Now: *The Grady Diet* encapsulates what has worked for me. Your duty, your loving duty to yourself, is to discover what works for you. Discover what's right and healthy for you.

There's no MD after my name. I'm no expert. No statistician. I'm just a guy who lost some weight. OK—it was a lot of weight. And a lot of people saw me and asked, "How did you do it?" A few even asked, reluctantly, "Did you lose that weight on purpose, or was it disease?" They still look at my old ID with a picture from seventy pounds ago and ask what my secret was. Recently, one bank teller, doubting my identity, nearly refused me a withdrawal.

Here's my advice to you. Take all received wisdom with the proper ear filters—including the Grady Diet. My friend, whatever new dietary practices you decide to adopt, do it gently. In the end, this book is simply one man's opinion, based on his dieting experiences. Throughout, I use the word diet in the sense of what we eat and how we live, but never in the sense of cutting back.

Now join me and your diet defender, Sparky Spaniel, for a great adventure in eating and living.

Grady Miller

Hollywood

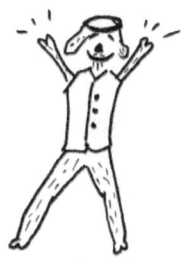

1. INTRODUCTION:
Love Yourself First

HAVE YOU EVER WONDERED what would happen if one of these authenticity-craving, showboating actors had fattened up for a movie role, in the true spirit of The Method, and then was later unable to shed the stage flab? Pretty funny, huh? Me, Grady, I lived the answer in the flesh. In preparation for a lead role in an independent movie, the director suggested I put on some extra weight. "Be a 'Method Larry,'" he said, referring to my character.

I heeded the director's suggestion with gusto. I deliberately threw myself into gaining thirty pounds, feasting on beer, pasta and Mexican pastries and fattening up for the role of sociopathic

Larry. As a veteran of different diets and training methods, I was confident I would know what to do so the pounds would melt away once the movie was complete and, at first, thanks in part to Cupid, everything was going according to plan. Two months after filming ended in Memphis, and the avoirdupois acquired for my movie role of Larry was no longer required, I asked the most important question of my life, "Would you marry me?" She said "yes," and in the weeks before my wedding, spurred by vanity, I slimmed down admirably before getting into my hat and tails.

Midnight Tacos

My fiancée also deserved credit for helping me to slenderize. She introduced me to **Fit for Life** by Harvey and Marilyn Diamond, a book I recommend for its emphasis on fruits and vegetables and, moreover, its passion about nutrition's role in enabling us to lead our most active, creative lives. **Lighten Up Now:** *The Grady Diet* embraces the core principles of this masterpiece, while simplifying it and taking it further.

Every country and culture has its nutritional pitfalls and socially sanctioned splurges. In Mexico, where I lived for nine years, there were midnight tacos and marathon Sunday family dinners. My in-laws' idea of a workout was sitting around the Sunday table and talking about going on a diet. The fact is, when the reality of marriage set in, my newly acquired slimness didn't stand a chance. Despite introducing me to this key book, my wife had her own eating habits, conditioned by Mexican culture and upbringing. She came from a family of restaurateurs and the daily after-school question wasn't, "What did you learn today?" It was, "What did you eat today?"

Midnight tacos really got under my skin. On a nightly basis. Being tempted by *carne asada*, while not hungering for it, made my flesh crawl. I would resolve to eat nothing and then suffer the indignity of having my defenses gradually broken down by the succulent smell of sautéeing beef and spicy pork, the nudges of my wife and the social pressure to give the taquero my business. However, to consume tacos at that hour, albeit delicious ones, washed down by the requisite ice-cold Coke was to be filled with self loathing. In my case, midnight tacos and marriage conspired to bring my post-Larry weight to new heights. I was tipping the scales at 232.

Gains and Pains

My first dieting experiences, as a teen, left me with a preference for going to bed on an empty stomach. The adage, "everything you eat after dinner turns to fat," encouraged this habit. An appreciation for hunger reinforced it: bless hunger that gives food its savor. The next meal after waking is called breakfast, get it? Breaking a fast. A period of non-eating, interrupted. You get out of bed with a snap, a spring you don't have when you've been digesting greasy animal flesh and corn masa all night long. If, on the other hand, you have long been a night snacker and are un-used to denying your mouth food after a certain hour, you may well imagine you'll be famished in the morning, but it's just phan-tom thinking. In the morning when you really, truly get the new day started, you'll find your five senses awakened and your ap-petite easily satisfied.

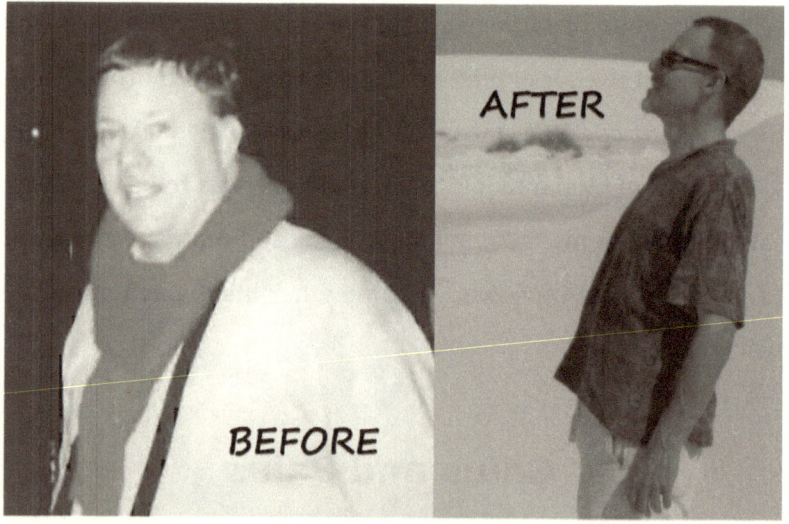

When life took me to Los Angeles, the Mecca of Cinema, I soon found myself in the heart of the movie business, managing a movie theater on Sunset Boulevard. It wasn't acting, but it had

great fringe benefits: popcorn galore, smothered in melted butter, nachos and a non-biodegradable yellow ooze that passed for
cheese sauce, and plenty of Dr. Pepper, Coke, and root beer. For a
treat we'd crack open a Toblerone for the staff, not to mention
Lindt Swiss chocolate, and Goobers, the toffee-coated peanuts
that Quentin Tarantino favored. All these goodies served to keep
me in size 38 pants as well as feeding a fleshy, unwanted part of
me that protruded over my waistline. To boot, I'd developed
chronic acid reflux which is a fancy term for heartburn. Under any
name, it's a painful phenomenon that is as hard to explain as love
for those who haven't experienced it. Suffice to say, the digestive
plumbing in my chest mocked and mimicked so many coronary
aches and twitches that when the "Big One" comes I shall be
blissfully unaware, chalking it up to "heartburn."

This time, when I decided to lose the weight accrued from the
movie theater, midnight tacos, and the movie role, I was motivated
not by teen anxiety or wanting to show off at a wedding or class
reunion. More than anything, it was a lark. I simply wanted to feel
better and gently improve my body. The weight-loss process
started from a place very OK with myself. That made all the difference: to initiate the process in a state of ease. I considered
myself in decent enough shape, and would have laughed if you
had accused me of being fat, though the camera and the scales
told a different tale.

The First Step

I started doing morning exercise. What André, an auto body-shop guy, told me about switching his workout from 10 at night to first thing in the morning, before breakfast, made so much sense. The morning exercise raised my spirits, and I gently slimmed. Over nine months I lost a couple belt loops and you could measure my past waistline by the shiny grooves the buckle left on my leather belt.

That first step—exercising before breakfast—was the most important. What's cool about first steps is that they always generate a second step and a third. So the outlines of a plan developed. It was an amalgam of techniques picked up from many sources: TV, friends, books and self-discovery. I picked up the "eating-only-at-mealtimes" from a TV appearance by Jack LaLanne, father of the modern fitness movement. Fit and feisty, he was then pushing ninety and still a vivid advertisement for the healthy living he preached. I confirmed the practice of sticking to mealtimes from a fellow theater manager who had been thin his whole life.

When you look at somebody who is in good shape—who embodies what you want to be—observe carefully. Take note, study their habits and emulate them; at the same time, cut yourself some slack from the get-go. Realize that these model people are the sum total of *years* of good habits and behaviors, formed and reinforced one at a time.

Real Benefits

The Grady Diet is not about losing 30 pounds in 30 days—though that is something you can do. It is about taking two years, or three, to become what you want to be, and learning to cultivate the practice of good habits, which will serve you for a lifetime. You'll be amazed how adopting these habits will benefit both your physical well-being and your pocket book. Here are just a few of the benefits of the Grady Diet:

> ➢ **Exercising at home saves gym fees**

> ➢ **Eat better and cheaper on fruits and veggies**

> ➢ **Feel better immediately**

> ➢ **Increased energy**

> ➢ **Avoid calorie counting**

> ➢ **Have more fun**

> ➤ **Greater overall health**

> ➤ **The probability of longer life**

Set yourself up for contentment, and start enjoying the benefits. You *do* eat better and *cheaper* when adopting the Grady Diet: fruits and veggies have greater nutritional value and are cheaper than most packaged, processed foods. Chances are, you will immediately feel better; you will notice your mood measurably improves the first day you start doing morning exercise. And once you discover that laughter equals exercise, you can start to have more fun. Also, avoid the hassle of calorie counting and frequent weighing. Your overall health will likely improve, and your blood pressure and dental bills will probably go down. Your teeth, once menaced by sugared sodas and the residue of processed foods, will cease to be a haven for caries-breeding muck, as they chew more fresh fruits and veggies.

I can vouch for the health benefits of the practices outlined here. Before the Grady Diet, my weight was 232 pounds, and my blood pressure was 120/80, which is considered the threshold for heart disease risk. After the Grady Diet I weighed 140 pounds, and my blood pressure had gone down to 99/66. My doctor said I had an "athlete's blood pressure." Wow! It was the first time in my life the word "athlete" had ever been applied to me in a positive context.

Chronic heartburn had long been a health problem for me, causing physical pain and affecting my mood. Every time I saw the doctor or pharmacist it was a nagging condition for which I sought relief. They usually recommended an antacid tablet; one doctor even recommended that I limit my consumption of fruit. None of them ever told me to simply try not eating between meals.

With the dietary changes described in **Lighten Up Now: *The Grady Diet***, the crippling heartburn drifted away. The pain I lived with for years now seems unreal as somebody else's nightmare. It takes an effort to remember the corrosive ache in my chest and remind myself what a dream it is to live today the Grady way.

The Grady Diet isn't about dogma, either. It's about being freed from the guilt mentality of calorie counting, developing the practice of new habits, and knowing that there's no sin other than failing to be OK with yourself and learning to accept yourself as you are. Armed with this knowledge, may you steadily cultivate love and patience toward yourself.

Once you get your habits down, if you're doing it 60% of the time that's good. Look at it this way, even 30% adhering to a healthier routine is infinitely better than zero percent.

Jack LaLanne said he felt proud whenever he fulfilled his promise to never eat between meals. Reading between the lines, this means even Superman was tempted. I dare say he didn't always manage to go without a nibble between meals—but most of the time. Nothing is "always." Set yourself free from always. Don't beat yourself up on those occasions when you break your personal diet code—they too will pass. Set your sights on practicing your new habits *most* of the time.

The Grady Diet is finally about tolerance for oneself. It's an evolution.

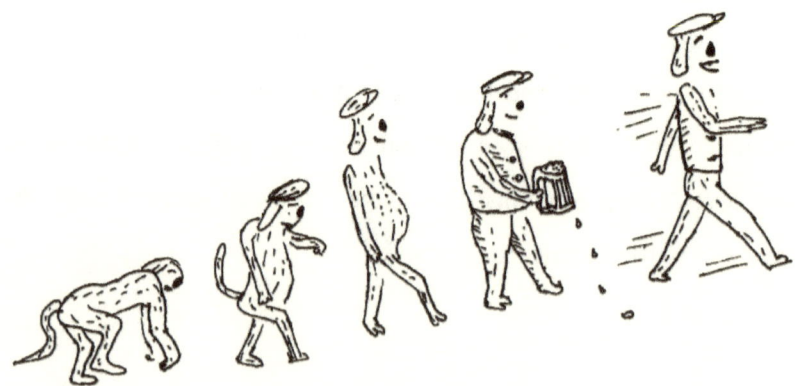

You know the first four letters of evolution are *love* backwards. So. . .

Love evolution
Love your body
Love yourself

Starting from that place of comfort with who and what you are, cocoon yourself in okayness. And start the change today.

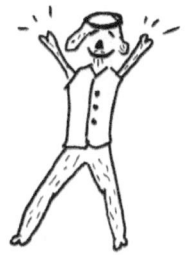

2. AFTER:

From fat to emaciated in 30 days

IN THE MONTHS before the cameras rolled, when I was chosen to play the lead sociopath in an independent movie shot in Memphis, Tennessee, the director casually suggested that I gain thirty pounds. (Only years later did he reveal that this had been said in jest.) The fact is, the director's wish was my command, and this was the inception of the Grady All-Beer Gaining Diet.

Little did I know that this extra weight acquired for my movie role would overstay its welcome and spawn the quest for a new way of living, eating, and managing my weight. Eight years after the cameras stopped rolling, I was left with a 38-inch waist, and today it's down to 31 inches. I lost in the range of sixty pounds in one year, and another ten over the next couple of years. What *was* my secret?

The tenets of the Grady Diet are presented here in the form of common questions and my answers.

How do I start?

Number one: Start from the place of "I'm OK just the way I am." This relieves the pressure and hair-pulling unhappiness and frustration associated with dieting.

Number two: Exercise in the morning, first thing. Get stretching and moving before you have a chance to become aware of your hangover. Your exercise time doesn't have to be long at all. For example, I have gradually developed a 20-minute routine of yogic stretches, sit-ups and leg lifts. You can walk for 20 minutes before breakfast, if you like. It's that simple.

People who exercise later in the day end up burning the calories from the food they have eaten. Exercising on an empty stomach burns the body fat directly before there is a new influx blood sugar in the veins. *This lifestyle change alone may be all you ever need to gently bring yourself to the perfect weight.*

So far you haven't told me anything about actual diet or food at all.

OK, here are my BIG FOUR dietary practices:

1. Eat only at mealtimes.

2. No beverages during meals. (Liquids slow down the digestion process by diluting the digestive juices.)

3. Fruit before noon. (This I now apply four weekdays, the other days are for reserved for eggs and hotcakes.)

4. Plenty of vegetables the rest of the time. Boiled, steamed, baked, sautéed, and fresh—especially in salads.

Anything else?

Yes, and it's a simple one. It's something your mom told you. **Eat with your mouth closed.** The practice of closing your mouth lends awareness to eating. You slow down, chew the food better. The saliva gets a head start on breaking down the food, as you enjoy the flavors and textures. Instead of shoveling it down, in a mechanical race to get it inside your belly, you awaken the senses and savor the joy of food.

Does eating only at mealtimes mean you are limited to three meals a day?

No. It means stick the best you can to mealtimes you've chosen. Maybe you're a person who eats five times a day. Fine. Set your five times and stick to them.

What if I get invited to eat during a time of day that doesn't coincide with my regular mealtime?

By all means, accept the invitation. The chance to socialize and share a meal takes precedence over your usual routine. You can exercise your dietary choices during the meal. And afterward, you have the opportunity to practice moderation: you may decide to eat lighter at the next mealtime.

One of your principles for losing weight is fruit before noon. What if I work the graveyard shift?

If you work graveyard or are a bon vivant who wakes up at the crack of noon, here's what you do. Consume fruit during the first four or five waking hours of the day.

Is there anything you won't eat?

Bread and other starches I usually shun. Put it this way: when I'm having rice, say, or pasta, it will be accompanied by a big salad or cooked vegetables, or both. When I adopted this practice of avoiding starches, I became slimmer. In fact, a number of people I know who were chubby and then, when I'd see them a year later, looked like movie stars, share this one common denominator: avoiding starches.

Also, reducing bread and starches is exactly the opposite of what I did to gain weight for the movie role when I gorged on beer and bread. Now the cinnamon swirls and Mexican pastries, which were a mainstay in the gaining diet, have also gone by the wayside.

But is there anything you absolutely won't eat?

Potato chips. Breaking up with Laura Scudders was hard to do.

Potatoes are a vegetable. Can I eat as many potatoes as I want?

Good question! I basically look at a baked potato as a slab of bread. Ditto mashed potatoes. It is preferable to stay away from these foods. However, here's how I deal with being offered a baked potato at a friend's house. If somebody has gone to the trouble of making a baked potato, done up with chives and all the good stuff, I will build a meal around it and make the potato the centerpiece. I will enjoy it and make sure that it goes hand in hand with ample vegetable portions.

In that kind of situation, being offered the baked potato, how do I handle the main course?

You get to practice saying two beautiful words that sometimes get a little rusty from underuse: NO THANKS. That's one alternative. Or you can accept the main course being served and say no thanks to the baked potato.

What about beer and other alcoholic drinks?

I'll have my beer or martini preferably half an hour before meal-time.

Do you ever have a beverage with your meal?

On rare occasion, when I can't get my water-rich vegetable fix I will have a beverage. Say it's a dry, impossible-to-swallow slice of roast. Then I will drink something, preferably water. Remember when confronting the choices of juice, soda or coffee, there's always the unspoken choice: clear, pure water.

What if I have a constant need to hop on scales and check my weight?

Don't bother keeping a bathroom scale around the house. Then you won't be tempted to the daily rush to judgment about the status of your diet. Also, losing the scales frees you from a cycle of guilt and recrimination that is perpetuated every time you see that needle creep onto an undesired number.

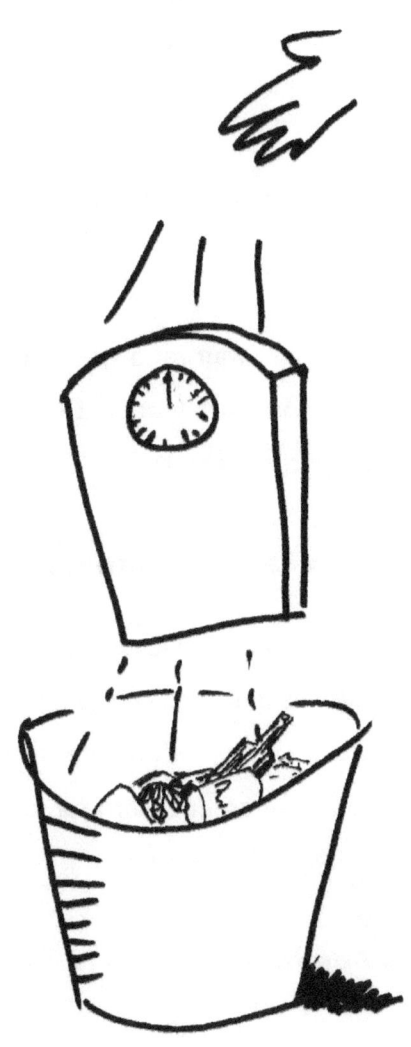

How can I tell how I'm doing on my weight if I don't have scales?

Look at how your clothes fit. Pay attention to your belt loops. Let your eyes tell you how you're doing, not a bunch of numbers between your toes.

As for calorie counting, don't even think about calorie counting. Free your brain.

If you must weigh yourself, wait for a visit to the doctor's office. Or use the scales when you are visiting a friend's house. I once used the scales at a recycling center!

What's wrong with calorie counting?

It leads to perverse beliefs about nutrition. Namely, the belief that something low in calories is a good choice because it will lead to thinness; that model thinness, which our society places on a pedestal. It leads to coffee and popcorn for lunch, and spurning an avocado because it's high in calories.

What else can I do to maintain a healthy weight?

Carefully watch what comes in your mouth and out of your mouth. That is, refrain from ridiculous assertions about food—i.e. after that piece of forever strawberry cheesecake, "I'll starve myself all week." Or "This will be the last piece of dessert I ever have." Such thoughtless phrases amount to threats against yourself and water the weeds of food mania.

Also, it is preferable to refrain from telling others how you may have lapsed and gone "off the wagon." First and most importantly, you're being unkind to yourself, tattling on yourself. Belittling yourself in the eyes of others. Nothing is gained.

Furthermore, should you confide in a gossip monger, you are being unkind to countless others. Many other people, who you may not even know personally, are earnestly striving for what you are striving for: to manage their weight. Hearing about your lapses from another person can negatively influence those who seek a better way to live and eat, and give them permission to slide. Be kind to yourself and everybody. Don't blab about your diet.

How long will I have to wait to see results?

A couple weeks should be enough. Maybe your pants will feel loose or you'll notice a change in the mirror. I counsel taking it easy and pursuing long-term results. You can do morning exercise, and continue to eat your old way. The change will become obvious as the months pass.

Or, if you are seeking more rapid weight loss, you can stick diligently to the BIG FOUR:

—Eat only at mealtimes

—No beverages during meals

—Fruit before noon

—Lots of veggies the rest of the time

Do these, plus **morning exercise** and a **moratorium on breads**. The results will be dramatic. Perhaps shockingly so.

Please take it easy, even if you do have a class reunion in two weeks. Befriend the mirror to monitor your face and body and see that you don't cross the line from supple to gaunt, as you slim down.

All right, I have adopted these practices, and the pounds have melted away. My friends and colleagues proclaim it in envious admiration. But what do I do about family members, who are afraid I'm sick?

These are the people who bugged you as a kid about your weight and bequeathed you with a problem, when in fact there was no problem. Now they accuse you of eating "rabbit food" and urge you to see a doctor. They really want it both ways. They want to insult you and sow insecurity, whether you're gaining or losing.

So they're to blame for my weight problem?

Not really. In the end, it's up to you whether you choose to listen to what motivates you or what devastates you. It's up to you.

Carefully choose the words you decide to listen to and the words you take to heart. You know, everyone has a right to feel good about themselves. Use your ears wisely to defend that human right. It doesn't matter what people say—family members especially. What matters is what you choose to believe.

And a sense of humor helps. Learn to laugh at others' ridiculous assertions, as well as your own. Indeed, 100 laughs equals ten minutes of exercise. So if you feel compelled to count something, start counting the laughs.

It will help both your body and outlook to discover laughter where you once found only hurt and anger.

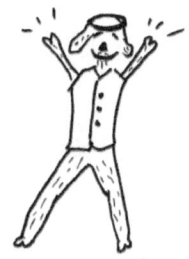

3. BODY-CHANGER:

The Importance of Morning Exercise

ANDRE RUNS A BODY SHOP in North Hollywood, where I had a dent taken out of my Toyota. As it turned out, André repaired much more than my car.

He was in stellar shape, not an ounce of fat on his perfectly toned and proportioned body. What was *his* secret? He told me that he used to exercise late at night, after work. His shape didn't improve. Then a professional trainer told him to exercise first thing in the morning, after waking up.

Exercising before you eat anything—the trainer told André—burns the fuel stored in the body's fat. If you exercise later in the day, after eating, exercise burns the blood sugar from the food you've already eaten during the day.

This blew me away. And it is worth repeating: *If you exercise later in the day, after eating, exercise burns the blood sugar from the food you've already eaten. Exercising in the morning, first thing, directly burns body fat.*

The moment I heard this, I adopted exercise in the morning.

The outward results were obvious during the first several weeks. My clothes became looser, and people commented how well I looked. Inwardly, from day one, morning exercise changed how I *felt*. My body was more limber and my mood, upbeat. When I fail to exercise in the morning, I can feel the difference: previously unfelt pains manifest themselves in my bones and muscles, and I catch my body being more sluggish and my mind more on edge.

Today, morning exercise helps me feel better and more resilient throughout the day, and it helps keep me in shape. Morning exercise is like an insurance policy for happiness; it generates pride in having already accomplished something at the start of each day. Further, it is a corrective during times of feast and celebration. So,

Morning Exercise

André repaired not only my car's body; he helped repair my own body and gave me a major tool to maintain it.

Trust me, you will be bowled over when you realize that morning exercise is as close to the one slimming secret as it comes. You can stop reading this book right now, start doing exercise in the morning, before you have had a single bite of breakfast, and claim for yourself the power to achieve the body you desire.

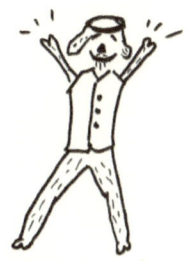

4. 100 Laughs:
Making it, faking it, doing it

AT THE BEGINNING of the full spectrum of laughter—which spans giggles, titters, chuckles, snickers, cackles, chortles, belly laughs, guffaws and side-splitting laughter—there is a noiseless snort that, although it emerges from deep within the chest, almost registers as silence, and that, too, is laughter. Then again, there are evil laughs, nervous laughs, angry laughs, tender laughs, and sad laughs. It's all laughter. . . and exercise.

The average child laughs 300 times a day; the average adult 17 times. Children who laugh 300 times a day are surely not connoisseurs of humor, demanding that everything be "really funny." They are proof that laughter is a reflex we are all born with, and it diminishes over time, like the moistness of our eyes (which incidentally, laughter helps restore).

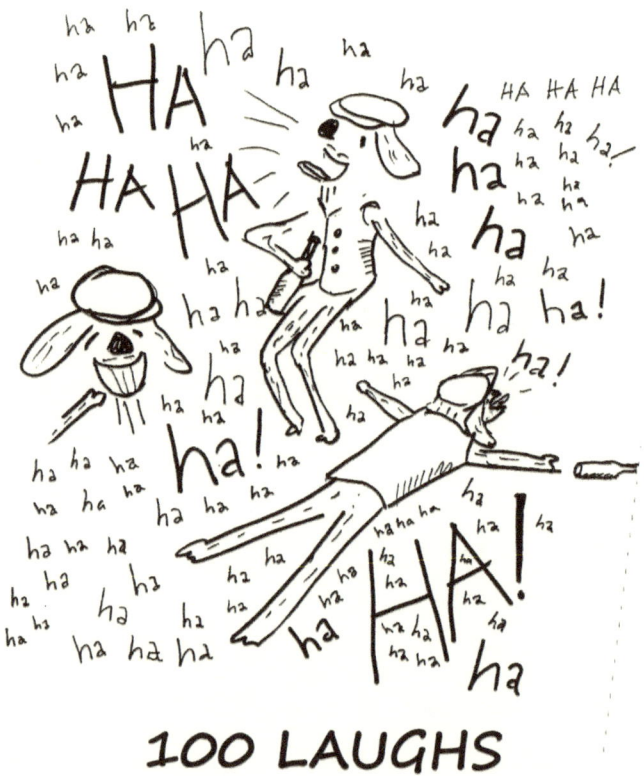

100 LAUGHS

Laughing gives your body a full workout. Try one minute of sustained laughter; believe me you feel it. Laughter involves muscles in the diaphragm, abdomen, lungs, legs and back, as well as the face. Some people even wave their arms when laughing. One hundred laughs, about a minute of continuous laughter, equals ten minutes of exercise, according to Dr. William Fry, the Stanford University professor emeritus who has spent a lifetime studying the effects of laughter on the mind and body. To start enjoying the calisthenic benefits of laughter, here is a simple method: **fake it**. Get used to the idea of faking it. Since your body can't tell the difference between real and simulated laughter, by faking it you will immediately start enjoying the phenomenal benefits. The first step to your 100 laughs a day is making and faking laughter. Don't wait for something knee-slappingly funny to happen. Get in the conscious habit of voluntarily laughing. Don't be shy. You can do it. A laugh doesn't have to be big or spontaneous. But there is a gaping difference between being told laughter is "good for you" and really doing it on a daily basis.

Dr. Madan Kataria is a physician who founded laughing clubs in India. His brainstorm came one 4 a.m. while researching an article he was writing on the medical benefits of laughter. The funny thing is, doing this research made him realize that he didn't laugh much and didn't have a very good sense of humor. Hence, the idea to form a laughing club, where people could "laugh over nothing at all." The first laughing club met at a Mumbai park in 1995, and clubs soon started sprouting up in other cities. The laughter quickly spread past India's borders, and in a few years the movement, popularly known as laughter yoga, had circled the world.

"You don't need any sense of humor to laugh," Dr. Kataria has declared in a CNN interview. "You don't need to be happy in order to laugh. In fact, when you laugh, you develop your OWN sense of humor. You develop joy within yourself."

Even infants deprived of sensory input giggle at the age of two months, which demonstrates humor is not a requisite for laughter. A study, conducted on blind and deaf newborns in Chicago in the 1950s, showed children spontaneously smile at around a month old, unrelated to the presence of anybody, and they giggle at two months. Laughter is, in Dr. Fry's words, "inherent behavior that is our heritage as human beings."

Now mental health professionals recommend "laughter therapy," which means laughing at things usually considered off-limits for mirth. This technique is a major addition to the arsenal of laugh-creating ploys. A funny approach to something really "serious" or embarrassing is a surefire way to get laughs—if only the nervous laughs of those listeners who think, "I can't believe I'm hearing this." The idea is to recognize a rich lode of laughter in what is often deemed "no laughing matter."

My Uncle John is an example of someone who did this intuitively. He had a great infectious laugh, a kind of a gasping wheeze honed by cigarette smoking, that so routinely punctuated his jokes, stories and patter, it brought mirth wherever he went. Well, Uncle John poked fun at a most unlikely topic: his stroke. He told the story about when he keeled over on the front lawn and couldn't move or speak, due to the stroke, from which he recovered to tell the tale complete with funny faces and sound effects.

Indeed, a considerable number of those who survived World War II death camps attributed their survival to an ability to laugh during the worst of times. In his memoir of Auschwitz, *Man's Search for Meaning*, Viktor Frankl writes, "Humor was another of the soul's weapons in the fight for self-preservation. It is well known that humor, more than anything else in the human make-up can afford an aloofness and an ability to rise above any situation, even if only for a few seconds."

Laughter frees us from the tyranny of reality and it also forms a bond. Laughter, as Victor Borge said, is the shortest distance between two people. I chart my own progress noting the things that make me laugh today that used to upset me. The difference between the funny side and suicide is all a matter of perspective.

So get to work. Whether you choose to fake it or take on a topic not normally associated with humor, start laughing at various times throughout the day to flex those abs. If you need inspiration to laugh, here are a few notions to prime your laugh-producing mechanism.

> **Catch yourself being serious. Have a chuckle.**

> **Look at those people on the subway, in the street with long faces, those sour-pusses in the office. You gotta laugh.**

> **When something happens that makes you think, "this really sucks." That's your cue: Time to laugh.**

> **When something works out perfectly, like you immediately find a parking place or your favorite soup is being served, laugh.**

> **Laugh, after a few judicious seconds, when plunged into despair over some-thing important you've lost.**

> ## Laugh when you find something lost that you were desperately looking for.

Laugh like crazy. People may think you are crazy. So what? Is that what happened to the child who once laughed 300 times a day for no reason at all? Did he or she get shamed into silence, fearful of being branded crazy? Laugh yourself to greater contentment as you give your body a thorough workout.

EXERCISE: Keep a Laugh List

Often, in adulthood, a toxic concentrate of worries crowds in on us at the end of the day, right before bedtime. Meanwhile, levity is so fleeting. We tend to blank out all the sparkling moments that produce giggles and chortles. The antidote to this is writing a "Laugh List" that helps to appreciate the lighter moments and monitor how often we are laughing.

Start keeping a list of brief descriptive notes about when and where you laughed today. The notes will help you remember the moments of laughter. It's great if you have five items at the end of the day to review. In the beginning you may have only one, and that's fine. Keeping a laugh list helps cultivate your capacity to laugh *and* to lighten up before you go to bed, so you can enjoy a really restful sleep.

At the end of the day your list may look something like mine:

> **7:20 am car didn't start – had to laugh. It was a loaner car from my mechanic.**

> **Mid-morning, nothing happening, decided to laugh.**

> **2:30 pm feeling down, timed 1 min. laughter (OK, I laughed only 30 seconds. A minute seemed forever.)**

> **9:30 pm at a dinner party, apple pie is served with ice cream – one woman is brave enough to turn it down; I am such a wuss. I caved in and had the apple pie. Gotta laugh at myself.**

> **11:15 p.m. YouTube video of Groucho Marx. Thumbs way up!**

After you practice faking laughter, it's OK to turn to the pros like Groucho Marx. Why not?

Chart your progress toward 100 or more laughs a day—which boils down to about a minute of laughter. Remember, Sparky's 100 laughs a day equals ten minutes of exercise.

You know, when you go back to the daily laugh list, there's an added bonus. You will hit on the occasional gem where something truly funny happened. Remember it, laugh again, imbue it into your memory, weave it into your conversation and make others laugh. There's no telling how far laughter will take you: not only be sexier and funnier, also feel better, lower your blood pressure and be smarter—all claims addressed in the next chapter.

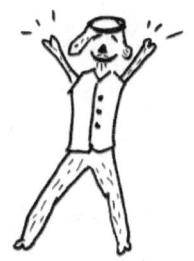

5. THE SEVEN STEPS

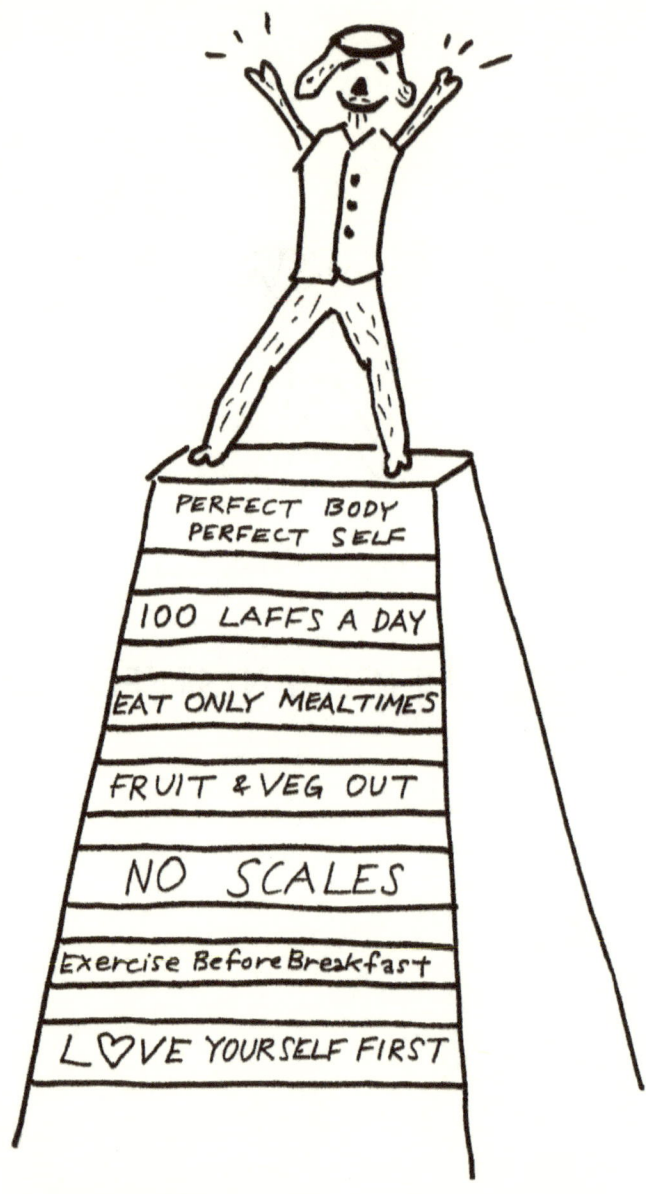

PERFECT BODY
PERFECT SELF

100 LAFFS A DAY

EAT ONLY MEALTIMES

FRUIT & VEG OUT

NO SCALES

Exercise Before Breakfast

L♡VE YOURSELF FIRST

SPARKY'S LADDER

THE FIRST STEP: Love Yourself First

WHEN YOU TAKE the first step onto Sparky's Ladder, you have committed to a new endeavor. You know how your house gets messy and dusty? Taking care of it is ongoing, a job that is never finished; so is improving yourself. The best attitude toward a never-finished job is knowing when to stop, so you don't go crazy. Do a little every day, then take pride in what has been accomplished.

Being OK with yourself is an ongoing job, trust me. I recently went to a party in Malibu and broke one of my cardinal rules: I ate too much. OK, I broke three rules: I ate too much, I drank while eating, and I nibbled tortilla chips and guacamole. It could easily have tailspinned into self-loathing, which is the epitome of being un-OK. Here's what I recommend doing when we feel yucky about transgressing our diet code: pinpoint something that you did better this time. For me, my accomplishment the night of the party was stopping at 7-Eleven at midnight, after the long drive back from Malibu to Hollywood, and buying a bag of sunflower seeds, instead of hot chocolate. Every time something like that happens, my diet defender Sparky barks his approval.

Find solace in that one little thing you did better, and move quickly on to today's assignment: learning to be OK with yourself. Now. Disliking something about yourself makes you weak—weaker still disliking something about yourself and starting a program of change based on self-dislike. It's like starting a foot-race on quicksand. Self-dislike can blossom into distress. Distress will inevitably take itself out on something or somebody else. Spare the world deplorable behavior where your issues become my hurt.

There is no worthier object of adoration than you—as you are. If you are reading this now, there is so much that is overwhelmingly right. You can breathe, feel, think, change. If there are things about yourself that you aren't crazy about, take action, but remove distress from the mix. Avoid becoming disgruntled or distressed for very long because the very instant you consciously reject distress and conjure that state of okayness, you are already treading the highest step on the ladder. You have already achieved the easy feeling of comfort in one's own skin, and that is the ultimate aim of all your fitness endeavors.

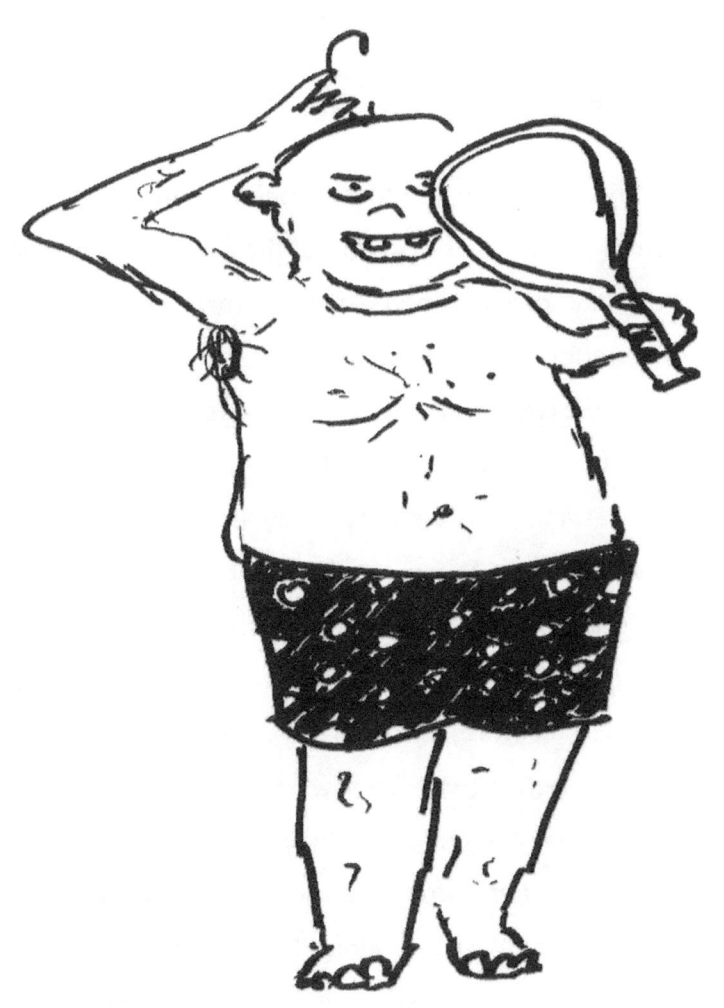

LOVE YOUR BODY. AS IS.

THE SECOND STEP: Morning Exercise

There's a very practical reason to exercise in the morning, before doing anything else. Get exercise out of the way and behind you. Later in the day, demands and activities crowd in and make it awkward to perform the panting and stretching involved in working out. The most compelling reason to exercise in the morning, of course, is that you will probably FEEL better, both physically and mentally. Aches and pains are kept at bay as the day progresses, and you are more likely to feel more resilient and upbeat. People who exercise later, aside from having to drop whatever they're doing, end up *burning the calories from the food they have eaten during the day*. In contrast, exercising on an empty stomach *burns body fat* directly, before there is a new influx of blood sugar in the veins. A study from Northumbria University (England), published in the *British Journal of Nutrition*, shows that people who have a pre-breakfast workout lose on average 20 percent more body fat. That's a clincher for those seeking to get in better shape.

But it gets even better. The findings of Australian researchers Megan Oaten and Ken Cheng in a study, published in 2006 in the *British Journal of Health Psychology*, suggest the far-reaching impact of exercise. Regular exercise has been shown to enhance the following:

—Exercise reduces stress

—Spontaneously causes people to start eating healthier

—Makes them less prone to distractions

—Improves people's spending habits

What more could you ask for? Exercise may be all you ever need to launch a successful program to improve yourself—your body and your pocket book.

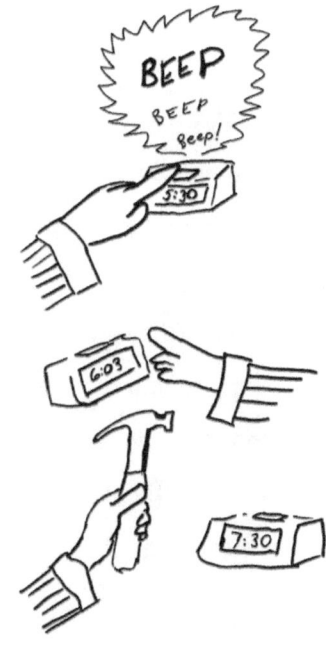

Morning Exercise

THE THIRD STEP: No Scales

Stepping onto the scale opens us to a direct assault on the carefully nurtured okayness and well-being that are vital to our journey up the ladder. Scales are the disapproving parent, the frowning authority. If an undesired number appears, we are scolded, and our thoughts and actions ricochet in harmful ways. If the scales go up, you think, "I'll skip breakfast," or you tell yourself, "I won't eat dessert for a week," and then, suddenly, you are imagining devious punishments for yourself and decreeing unrealistic behaviors that, when you fail to carry them out, produce ill-feelings and undermine self-respect.

If the numbers on the scale are going down, that's another story. You are happy. It reinforces your identity as a successful weight-loser, and you may brag to people, "I lost five pounds this week." The lower numbers may even give you permission to "splurge." Instead of encouraging the habits that got you to this point, it's turned a less healthy choice into a reward. You'll treat yourself to a piece of cheesecake because you lost five pounds. You may be calculating, "I lost two pounds this week, and this was only an eight-ounce piece of cake. I'm still ahead of the game," and yet, even as you are forking bitefuls of cheesecake, you are mentally connected to "the scale."

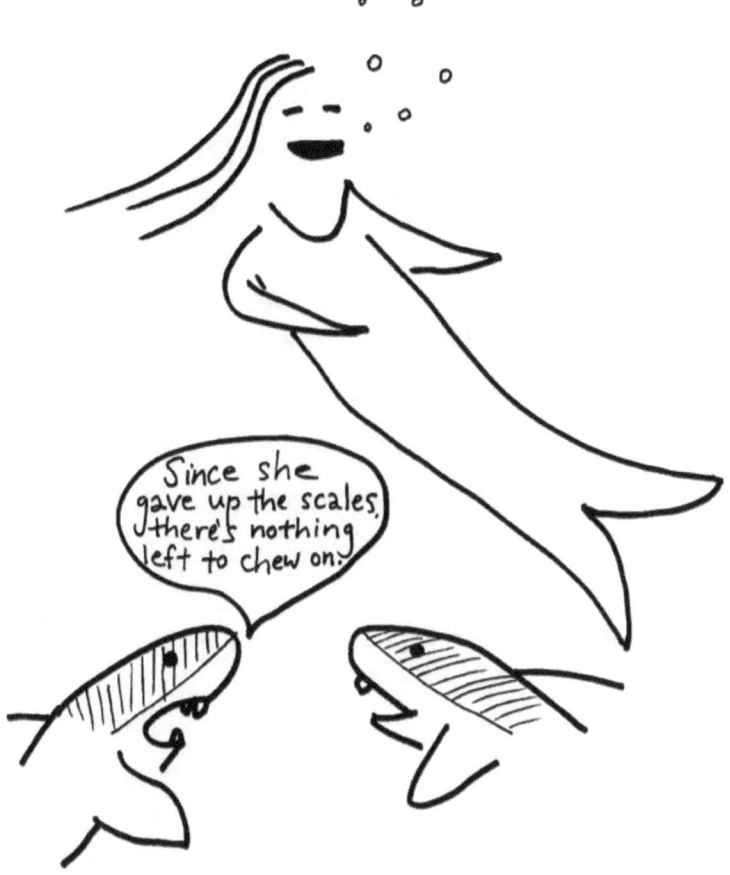

THE FOURTH STEP: Fruit and Veg Out

This is the fresh juicy crispy crunchy glorious good stuff that nature has produced abundantly. Cooked or raw, in soups, salads or smoothies, home-grown or store bought, purple, orange, green, yellow or red. Be generous. Give yourself as large a portion as you like. Be bountiful. Keep a fruit cornucopia on your table and vegetables in your fridge.

This is one of the few times I'm going to mention the C-word. Calories. Fruits and vegetables—the stuff that grows on trees or sprouts out of the ground—is low-cal, which is why we can eat them freely. Also, fruits and sweet vegetables, such as yams and carrots, are great for satisfying our sweet tooth.

Always welcome fruits and veggies onto your plate.

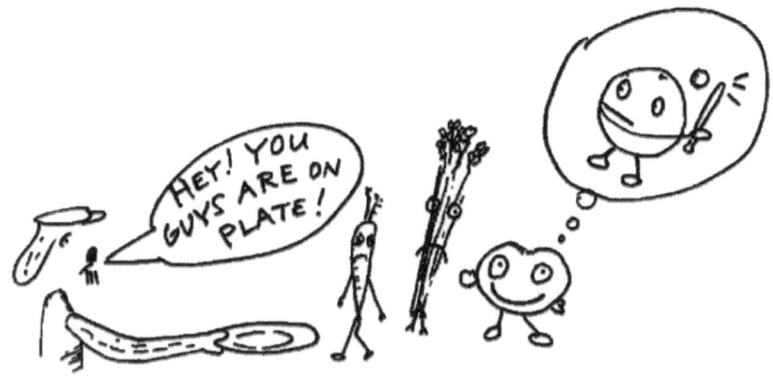

When you go to the grocery store, head straight for the produce section. Gaze in awe: what is pyramided in the aisles and appealingly arrayed in the tilted refrigerated section, beautifully free of packaging, signifies an investment in your well-being. Isn't it funny how every box of cereal has an exhaustive nutritional label showing vitamins and minerals, and detailing fat, carb and protein content? Here in the fruit and vegetable section we are left blessedly alone.

The produce section is nature's vitamin store! Fruits and vegetables are packed with vitamins and minerals. Obtaining these in their natural form, many nutritionists believe, is better than bottle vitamins. Two examples: Oranges are rich in vitamin C and calcium. Carrots are loaded with vitamin A, are beneficial for eyesight, even promoting night vision, and they're full of fiber. Many studies show that fruits and vegetables may protect the body against cancer and promote heart health. Onions and tomatoes have been shown to help prevent prostrate and liver cancer. Beets produce mood-boosting serotonin, one of the body's "feel-good" chemicals. The vitamin C and beta-carotene in spinach may help prevent Alzheimer's disease, and celery, according to some studies, decreases stress hormones and improves blood flow, thereby lowering blood pressure.

In the Grady Diet, fruits and vegetables are the counter-balance to other foods that don't come off a tree or out of the ground. If you are going to have a juicy steak or a piece of pizza, for example, make sure it's accompanied by a ton of veggies. It's that simple. And by a "ton" I mean a salad that fills a whole dinner plate and/or half a dinner plate full of veggies along with your main dish.

This practice is backed up by compelling chemical reasons. Fruits and veggies contribute to the body's internal balance between alkaline and non-alkaline fluids, produced by digestion. This is called the pH level. When the body's pH level is balanced it closely resembles water (neutral)—pure water produces neither alkaline nor non-alkaline fluids in the body. The body's optimal balance is just a shade alkaline. In this clear-water state the body is more likely to burn fat for fuel, and weight is likely to remain stable.

Keeping in the clear-water balance is also easy on the kidneys. When the body is breaking down steak or pizza or other foods that don't come out of the ground or grow on trees, it produces non-alkaline fluid (acid). The kidneys work overtime to remove this acid from the bloodstream, and it is released from the body as urine. When the diet is high in fresh fruits and veggies, the kidneys have less acid to remove.

Also, fruits and vegetables have a vital hydrating function, which goes hand in hand with the practice of drinking beverages a half hour *before* or *after* a meal, and not *during* it. By satisfying thirst, fruits and veggies facilitate being able to go without drinking, while eating, which in turn speeds our body's digestion.

In short, eating lots of fruits and vegetables will probably help you feel better and become slimmer. That's really all you need to know. Above all, eat fresh fruits and vegetables because they taste good—not just because they are good for you.

FIFTH STEP: Eat Only At Mealtimes

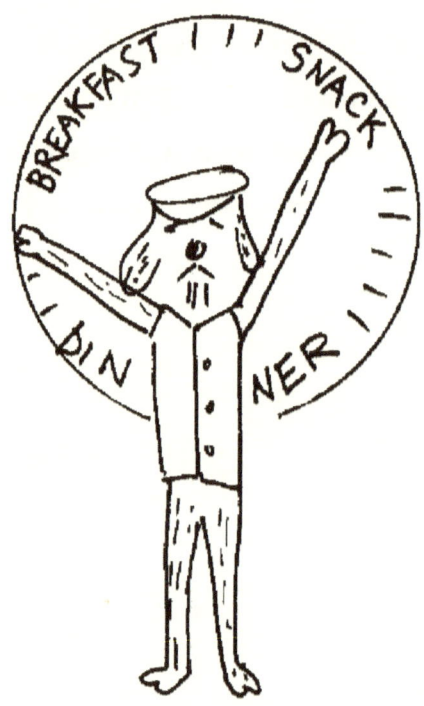

This is breathtakingly simple. If you are not munching all the time, you are going to be eating less. Your body will be doing more with less fuel, and this will enhance your shape. If you have three meals a day and a midmorning snack, set those as your meal-times. If you eat seven times a day, set the times for those.

Whatever plan you have, set the times and stick to them. When you respect the limits you've set for yourself, believe me, you will feel better. It will give you fuel and encouragement to continue up the ladder.

Indeed, I cannot stress how helpful it is to set limits and abide by them. The non-eating times are when we are active, living life, learning, and working. The non-eating times are also what make the times when we do eat special. Our hunger is sharpened, and we are grateful to break bread, even though with the Grady Diet we are more likely to break carrot sticks.

SIXTH STEP: 100 Laughs a Day

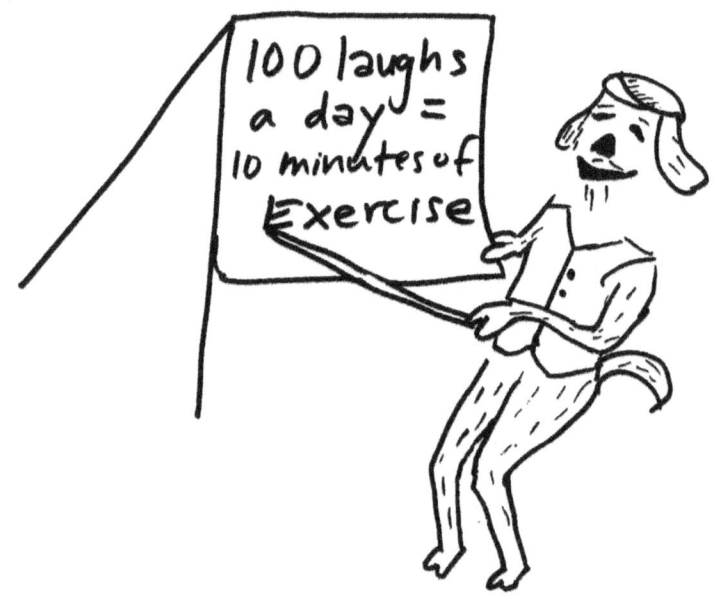

Soon as the myriad benefits of laughter for the mind and body soak in, you will immediately want to do two things: start faking laughter or get your butt to a comedy club.

Yes, laughing gives your body a full workout. Using muscles from the face to the legs, laughter involves the lungs, and the heart:

the pulse and blood pressure spike briefly, we breathe faster, causing increased oxygenation of the blood. Afterward, blood pressure decreases notably. In a study conducted on tech industry employees in India, a lasting decrease in blood pressure was noted after just three weeks of laughter yoga sessions. The sessions—seven in all—consisted of one minute of simulated laughter, followed by intervals of gentle stretching and deep breathing, repeated for 20 to 30 minutes. Blood pressure in the people who completed the seven laughter sessions lowered from 128/82 to 121/79. Meanwhile, the control group remained unchanged.

Laughter reduces the stress-producing hormone cortisol, and boosts pain-relieving endorphins—brain chemicals associated with the runner's high—demonstrated in research conducted by Dr. Lee Berk at Loma Linda University in California. Within the framework of brain plasticity (the new concept that the brain is still growing cells and capable of renewal), humor can actually make our brains bigger. A joke can reveal a new way of looking at things, illuminate a truth, exploit two meanings of the same word, or present something absurd. "There's something there that you haven't thought of before, something new, a discovery," says Dr. William Fry, whose pioneering research showed that 100 laughs equals ten minutes on a rowing machine. "It's an idea which you have not been the host of previously. As a result of that, you've set up a new network of neurons in your brain—these little cell structures which are in interconnection with all the other cell structures in the brain. You're having discovery, new connections are taking place, and the consequence of that—guess what?—your brain is bigger than it was a few minutes ago."

The lowdown: Jokes are barbells for your brain, so feel free to have an occasional stiff one, since you can always regenerate those dead brain cells.

7. Perfect Body, Perfect Self

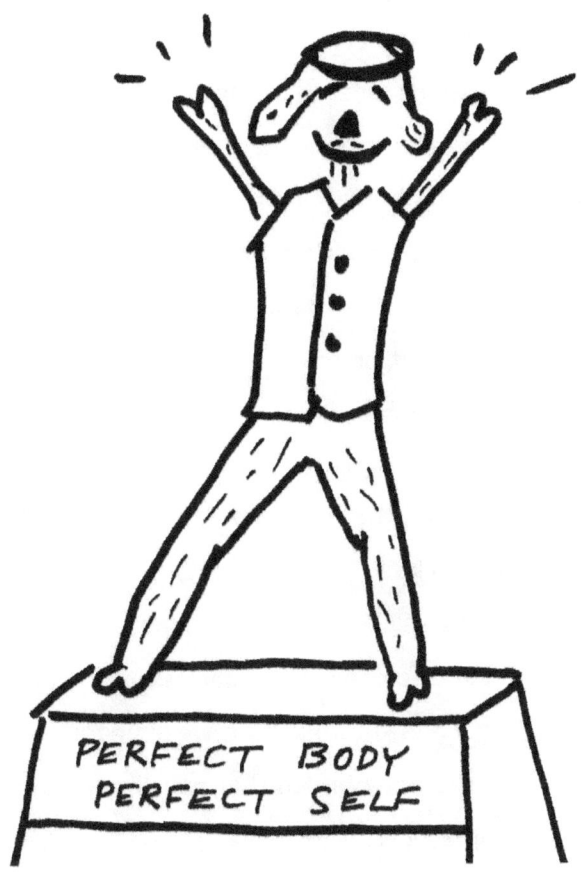

Fixating on the final seventh step will cause you to become obsessed and disgruntled. You may despair, *My perfect body and self are farther away than ever; look at me—my sagging arms, bulging belly and jiggling chins.* When you harbor this distress, you'll feel puky and tense inside. I know I do. Some people are so used to this feeling, it becomes normal for them; they feel like they are missing something when they lack this awful, stomach-tightening tenseness. Learn to be acutely sensitive to that nasty feeling aroused by disliking something about yourself; become as sensitive as one of these instruments whose needles jump when the earth trembles half way around the world. Become allergic to resentment against yourself or resentment toward any of your own physical traits that displease you.

Now that we have reached the final step—Perfect Body, Perfect Self—get ready for a "spoiler." You were pretty OK when you took the first step: Love Yourself First. You are perfect, you always were. And yet, as in the case of a good many lessons, there's a big gap between learning it and knowing it, between hearing about it and living it. So we constantly bridge that gap through reading, moment-by-moment practice, and exercises.

We have ended precisely where our journey began. T.S. Eliot wrote in *Four Quartets*:

The Seven Steps

We shall not cease from exploration
And the end of all our exploring
Will be to arrive where we started
And know the place for the first time.

We may stray. There may be lapses. But being OK with ourselves

is our home, our anchor, our unalienable birthright.

EXERCISES

EXERCISE #1   Instant OK-ness

Ask throughout the day: Right now am I listening more to my thoughts or my senses? Whatever the response, this will automatically hasten a balancing adjustment and help you gently come to your senses.

If you are listening to your thoughts and deaf to your senses—time to lighten up. Chin up, eyes and ears wide open. You are one deep breath from OK. Behold the movement of people, the play of sunlight, the screech of brakes, a baby waving from a stroller. If you are unaware of what is happening right now and here in front of your nose, adjust yourself away from thoughts to the senses: sight, sound, touch, taste and smell.

EXERCISE #2   Allergic to Un-love

This first step on Sparky's Ladder—being OK with yourself and your body—is so important. Let's do an exercise to prepare you and bring you to this step. Since it's easier and often more obvious to observe others, take a day or two to observe friends, family, and co-workers. Notice when they are being unloving and unkind to themselves.

It could be getting really upset about a stain on their clothes. It could be belittling themselves, albeit in a joking way ("I'm a terrible singer. I could never carry a tune.") or their body (not smiling for a picture because they are ashamed of their teeth); it could be letting a loved one's words ("You always ruin everything!") spoil the day or wigging out about something misplaced ("Where's my credit card? Somebody could be buying out the store. Holy cow, I better call the bank.") And, of course, look for examples of physical aggression against oneself, such as somebody pounding their fist on their forehead and saying, "I'm an idiot."

Be on the lookout for this harmful behavior in other people. Now here's your assignment: **Jot down ten examples of a person being unkind to themselves in word, thought or action.**

When you have listed ten examples of self-unkindness, look at them, study them. You are now going to put yourself on a total fast for these kinds of self-hating thoughts and disrespectful

behaviors towards yourself. Start identifying these un-loving behaviors in yourself and weed them out today. Replace these with
laughter and love.

EXERCISE #3   **Love List**

Use your imagination. Think of all the ways you can start loving
yourself both in your life and diet. What words can you use to
cheer yourself on? What deeds and habits can foster wellbeing?

Here are a few ideas for starters:

1. Loving yourself is looking in the mirror in the morning and
smiling.

2. Loving yourself is having something for breakfast, no matter
what you ate yesterday. Even if it's a single piece of fruit.

3. Loving yourself is knowing when to say, No thanks.

4. Loving yourself is forgiving yourself when you forgot to say, No
thanks, when you should have.

5. Loving yourself is giving yourself time and taking off your swea-
ter when it gets too warm. Or putting it on when it's cold.

6. Loving yourself is taking off a shoe and shaking it when there's
something inside that's irritating your foot.

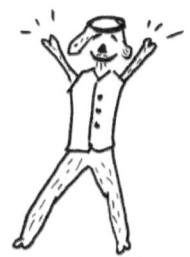

6. BEFORE:

From emaciated to fat in 30 days

THE GAINING DIET, conceived to prepare me for a movie role, can be summed up in two easy-to-remember words—anything goes. With a devotion proper for artistic creation, I ate everything I liked for two months, and with each mouthful of food and gulp of beer I was sculpting my movie character, Larry.

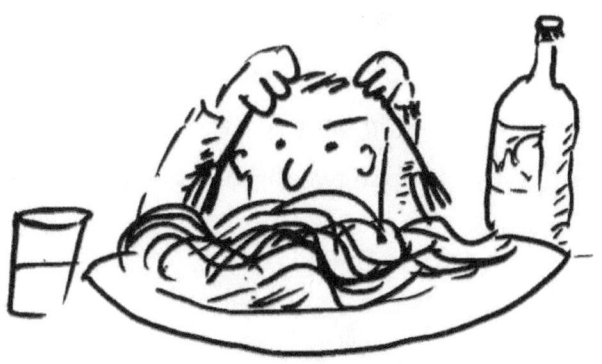

The diet had pedigree, for it was established in emulation of that chameleon-like method actor, Robert De Niro, who transformed himself for every role, especially for his portrayal of Jake LaMotta in *Raging Bull*, where he chose to put on real pounds instead of a fat suit.

De Niro had Italy, and the villages of Tuscany to roam, for his all-pasta diet during a break in *Raging Bull*, when he morphed from sleek young Jake to bloated old Jake. I had Mexico, for my all-beer diet. This country, which I called home for many years, is every bit Italy's peer when it comes to rib-sticking delicacies and kaleidoscopic flavors.

Breakfast was eggs scrambled with chorizo or bits of fried tortilla; sweet breads galore, conchas, doughy brown pig-shaped cookies, and flaky orejas wolfed down with acrid draughts of Nescafé. (Admittedly, prejudices about boozing before noon kept me from quaffing beer at breakfast.) For lunch, *tortas ahogadas* left my mouth on fire, and a nice Pacifico or Estrella put out the three-alarm blaze. In the evening, roasted chicken, lots of Kraft macaroni and cheese slathered in dairy butter—all accompanied by Fritos or potato chips and up to two caguamas—the equivalent of 64 ounces of Mexican beer.

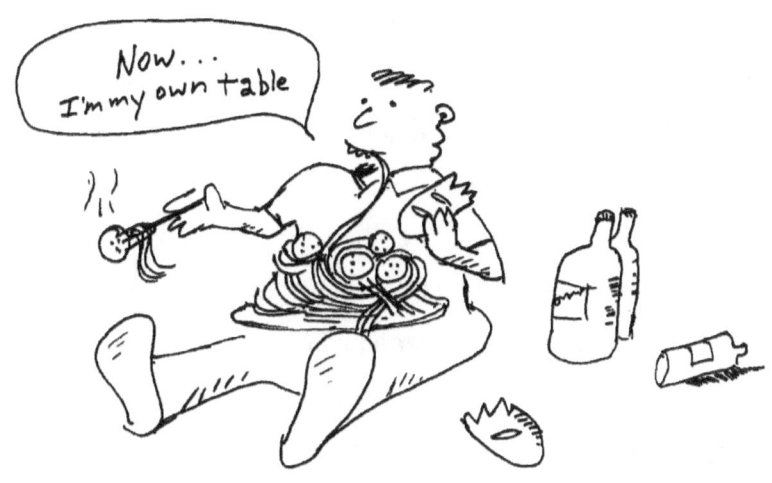

Gradually, I had to let my belt out, and strained my shirt seams. I accomplished this dietary feat by *becoming* the character I was playing. In a profound way, I *was* Larry Cartwright, prevaricating, beer-swilling, charming con-artist. Larry would never have given two hoots in a hollow about what he ate. He was the kind of guy to make goats look like picky eaters.

Filming progressed at a workmanlike pace throughout the summer in Memphis' malarial Overton Park, the movie's main locale. My mosquito bites had mosquito bites, and if I got tired of itching those red bumps there was plenty of poison ivy to go around. The weather gods had two thermostat settings: broiling swelter for grilling people during the day and then, after sundown, a rare climate splendid for grilling meat and drinking beer late into the night.

As August turned to September, fall turned the foliage brown in Overton Park, and filming suspended for eight long months. During this hiatus I could strictly adhere to the Grady Gaining Diet, for the sake of continuity.

To be truthful, the Gaining Diet could be termed an all-bread diet. German monks considered beer liquid bread and in ancient times brewed it as a supplement in times of fast. Mexico has a staggering assortment of bread (no less a gourmand than Orson Welles declared it the world's best), and a special bread is baked for most holidays. Day of the Dead boasts *pan de muertos*, which resembles a sugar-frosted, dough version of the San Onofre nuclear generating plants.

After the humongous Christmas repasts and posadas—the traditional serial parties leading up to December 25th—even the sixth of January, Three Kings Day, features a wreath-shaped sugar-frosted bread, crossed by red and green jelly strips, that contains a fingernail-sized doll representing the baby Jesus. According to tradition, whoever gets the doll in their piece of bread, is obligated to host a party on Candlemas, February 2nd (a.k.a. Groundhog Day). There is also an unwritten tradition that whoever gets the baby Jesus doll usually forgets to host the Candlemas party.

At Easter time capirotada appears in Mexican kitchens. It is a chewy Lenten bread pudding that surreally combines melted cheese, brown sugar, and hard crusty French bread. I really had to do a double take the first time I tried it.

All these remarkable breads helped contribute twenty or thirty pounds, according to the occasional drug store scale. (Remember: *whether you are gaining or losing*, it is far better to keep no scale in your home.)

My biggest thrill, after the long journey from Mexico to Memphis, was loping into the house of the director, after eight months of hiatus, and hearing the first words out of his mouth, "Perfect continuity." Now, this year, after seeing the amazing results of my new losing diet, the director exclaimed with devastating truth and wit, "You killed Larry!"

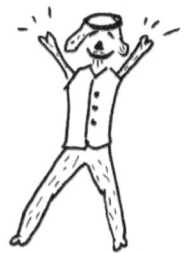

7. I'M NOT VEGETARIAN:
And a few more secrets

THIS BOOK STARTED as a series of tips I wrote down for a guy at the dry cleaners, who wanted to know the secret of my thinness when I brought in a pair of pants to be taken in. People kept asking for my secret. Over time, the tips became a comic essay with a sincere core, then a pamphlet, and finally, after many moons, it grew into the book you are reading. This slow germination has given me the gift of being able to ponder where I'm weak in practicing what I preach, and it has made me aware of several odd practices I actually do but didn't mention.

Any one of these "secrets" may provide just enough extra mojo to help you succeed in your new way of living and eating.

—Leave a little on the plate One small but very meaningful gesture is leaving a little on the plate. Through it, you are owning the choice to stop eating. And by leaving something on the plate, you're telling people and yourself: "There is always enough." Also, you are triumphing over the deeply conditioned belief in "clean up your plate"—which enfeebles our own innate ability to know when we've eaten enough.

I like my uncle's explanation for this practice best. One morning in the coffee shop, my dad asked my uncle why he always left something on the plate. "I don't know," Uncle John chuckled. "I guess I leave it for the angels."

—Practice Saying 'No Thanks' Simply say 'No thanks' gracefully when a person offers you something to eat that isn't right for you. Avoid the urge to narrate why you're saying 'No thanks.' For example, somebody offers you fresh fruit. Yet you feel no hunger; your stomach tells you so, and you know why. Just say 'No thanks,' and leave it at that. When you narrate what you previously ate (or overate), you create food villains and you turn others' generosity into villainy—which is a far more serious transgression than going off any diet. It messes with people's fundamental flow of giving. Better be free of all that and leave open the future possibility of guiltlessly enjoying once again the food that made you, on this occasion, say 'No thanks.'

—Segue out with fruit or nuts Say you had something massive and heavy, like a bagel slathered in cream cheese or a wedge of red velvet cake. Segue out with fruit or some nuts. Nuts bring the palate away from the sweet. And fruit, with its high water content, serves as a solvent. A zesty orange or some juicy ripe strawberries, for instance, refresh the whole body.

—Chewing gum Always a good choice during the periods of non-eating between mealtimes, chewing gum helps reinforce the practice of not eating between meals. I do recommend ditching the gum when you go on a date and those other times when you want to look your best or just plain sexy. Like my grandmother said, "Never dress up and chew gum."

—Out of sight OK, the best solution is not to have certain tempting foods around the house. Foods that call out to you, when you see them; they leap out and say, "Eat me." You may like to keep them around for a treat, or for a loved one, but put them out of sight, in a drawer or cupboard. When something is out of sight, you're much likelier to be free of its spell.

Likewise, prominently display fruit and vegetables. Their visibility is subtly training yourself to make fruits and veggies your default food choice.

—I am not a vegetarian There are people who must eat meat with every meal, there are fruitarians, who eat only fruit. Others extol eating raw foods and find it so healing. I embrace fruit and vegetables wholeheartedly, disengage from bread and other starchy foods, and eat meat moderately.

My yoga thinness and emphatic emphasis on fruits and vegetables lead people to falsely assume I am vegetarian. Early in the Grady Diet I went through nearly meatless seasons, and there were seasons of white meat—fish and turkey and chicken—and now the occasional steak. It's been an evolution.

—Many things work The dogma of the Grady Diet is to be free from dogmas. That's why you have diet books that minutely explore one facet of nutrition and demonize one food, or place another food on a pedestal. And these books can also contain useful things to learn and adopt. Be and stay open.

Everyone wants the one secret. The secret is: there is no one 'secret' but many secrets. What works is an amalgam; the notions come from many sources, constant observation, and the compost of statistics, which I use sparingly. My motto is keep it easy, brother and sister, you've already got enough distracting data coming at you. Simpler is better.

In being studiously non-scientific, I am free to present all my findings for effective practices and spare you all the statistical and nutritional blablabla. This is in tune with human nature, as I perceive it: we mix and match, learn by trial and error. This is the evolutionary fun of every day, truly the spice of life, to observe this grand experiment in progress.

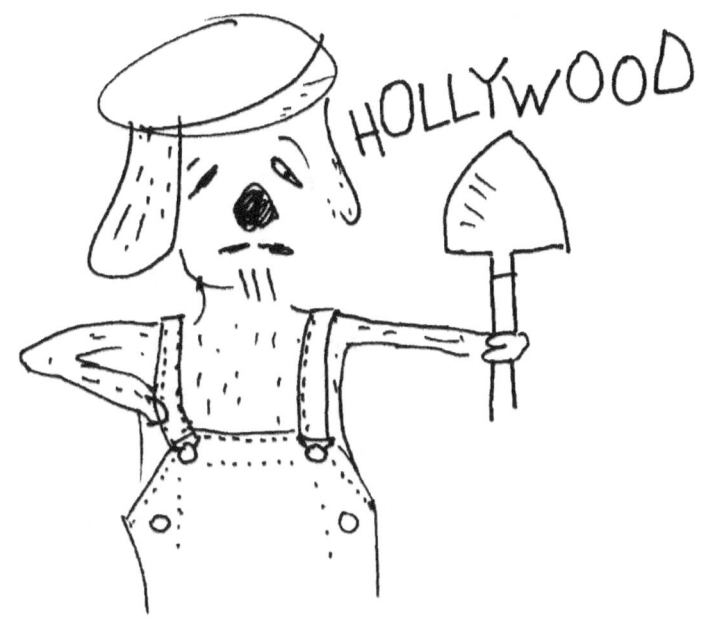

8. GROWING YOUR OWN:
Hollywood Style

WHO WOULD'VE THOUGHT that by schlepping my Adonic carcass to the mecca of tinsel, I would discover agriculture? Yes! It's Green Acres in reverse: kid from a small farming town in Central California comes to the big bad city, and becomes a farmer. Indeed.

Recharged by generations underneath a smothering skin of concrete and asphalt, the fallow Hollywood soil, once home to acres and acres of renowned orange groves, is just itching to become fruitful again.

Mine own eyes have seen the power of Hollywood soil. A dirty thumb needn't be endured, much less a green one. You just need to be there for the harvest. The fruit trees take care of themselves; they are organic in the purest and laziest sense—no spray, no irrigation, no sweat, and best of all, no label to peel off. When I finally decide to don bib overalls and chew on a straw all day, it will be solely a fashion statement. With the ease of a crop that virtually raises itself, the Hollywood farmer could wear a white tux into the field.

Last summer (growing season in farmers' parlance) was my first agricultural foray. I threw some seeds for butternut squash in a corner of my garden. It was late in the season, July, and still the clover-like leaves sprouted out of the ground. I thinned them out as the seed packet instructed. By late August one vine predominated and snaked around inside the fence, and yet bore no fruit until reaching the southern exposure at the other side of the fence: blossoms appeared and then the vine grew a single squash that reached full succulence in late September. The most mouthwatering, delicious squash ever to grace a semi-stick pan.

Extraordinary pride came from planting a single seed, watching it grow, and tasting the results.

Licking My Chops

Becoming a front-yard farmer has raised an awareness for the earthly elements—the sun and its direction, the precious water without which a plant can wither. Hitherto oblivious of the seasons, I now grasp their immense importance: in Hollywood, fall means oranges and avocadoes, spring, the slow-ripening tangerines, tomatoes start in August, grapefruit are year round thanks to the high branches which few people ever manage to pick. The sweet ripe yellow fruit remains tantalizingly on top while deep green clusters of new grapefruit form on the lower branches.

I'm licking my chops as the German neighbor lady's orange tree ripens, as the orb-laden branches turn from lime green to bright orange, and the tree makes good its promise of fleshy fruit that will fill a whole room with the invigorating smell of broken orange. Planted half a century ago by her daughter in a narrow space between cottages, the tree yields the sweetest navel oranges. Unlike the horribly bitter, face-scrunching peels of store-bought oranges, the mild rind of these Hollywood organics can be eaten.

The bounty of these resilient citrus trees is inexhaustible. Oranges, lemons, tangerines. As many grapefruit as I want: last year a non-profit harvested 318 pounds of grapefruit from the neighbor's tree after I'd had my pick for months. At least a hundred more pounds were left dangling on the tops of the branches.

The tangerine tree was the focus of a magical neighborhood event. Two neighbors joining to prune the tree spontaneously generated a whole Saturday afternoon in which a half dozen residents in our cottage court gathered to cut branches and harvest. Bag upon bag of the incredibly orange fruit, whose peel slips effortlessly off, was harvested. It was like Halloween meets a barn-raising, and for one chilly autumn afternoon we shared the magic.

A Big Lesson

We have vegetables, too. The lady who bought her cottage for $5,000 in 1940 has cherry tomatoes this year. The eye sharpens as new ones turn from a jaundiced green to bright lipstick-red almost overnight. They will rot on the vine before somebody picks them all.

These trees and plants teach a lesson in abundance, bringing forth prodigal bounty from the earth. In the natural order, one un-watched, unwatered tree produces more fruit than a single family can possibly consume. If we all enjoyed these fruits, we might be a bit more at ease about "putting something on the table." And taking advantage of neighborhood fruit will shorten our grocery lists, too. In front of my house Asian chile bushes now blossom, which augurs the arrival of fruit. I'll never buy a chile pepper again. And never again will grapefruit, oranges or tomatoes go into my grocery cart. And nothing ever will taste as good as something I grow myself, with a little help from the rich Holly-wood soil and the awesome Southern California sun.

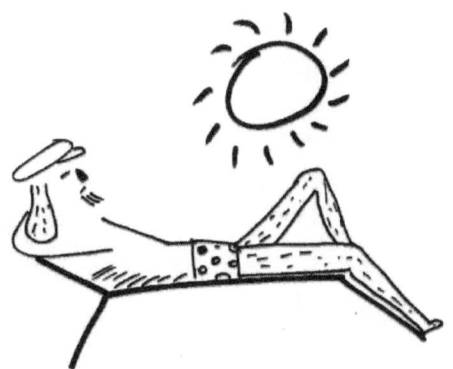

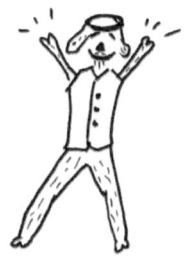

9. BACKWARD:

The Grady Story

I JUST SPENT a whole Sunday afternoon engrossed in a weird new pastime: hunting through piles of old snapshots to find the fattest, grossest, most bloated and porcine picture of me in existence. This peculiar activity turned out to be exhilarating.

You know how the ego zeroes in on a photo of yourself and says, Look at my zits, look at my double chin, and you exclaim, "That's an awful picture," oblivious to the 130 other people standing alongside you at the Miller family reunion? That's human nature: turning the spotlight on our own perceived defects, and suffering needlessly because of it.

Get this: I actually felt disappointment searching through these old photos because this or that snapshot showed me too slender. Or my winter scarf too successfully dissembled my double chin. Look, I needed a dramatic *before* picture to contrast with my dramatic *after* shot. In the end, I was glad for this added new experience. The search for the best fat shot brought me ever closer to the blissful realm of clear-sighted objectivity, and being OK with who I was and who I am.

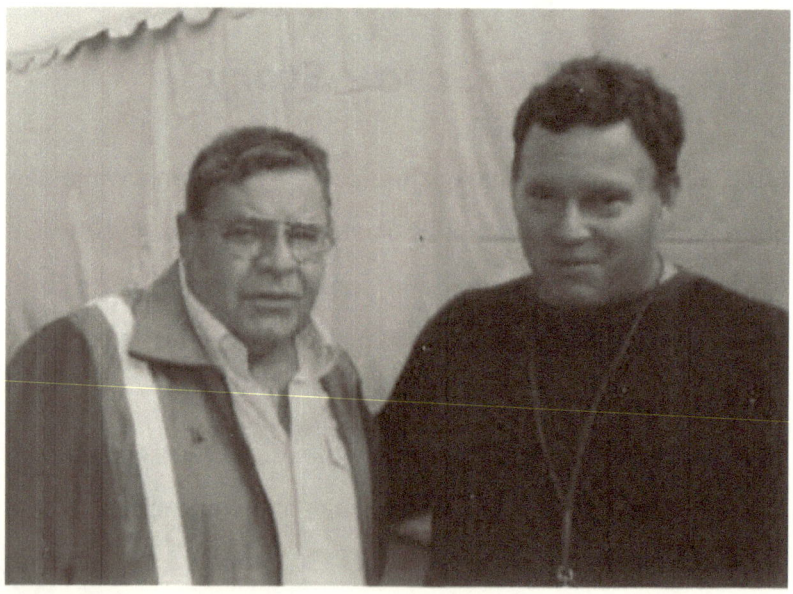

Two comic heavyweights compare girth. . . er, mirth. (Runner-up 'Before' shot)

I was not always so loving and lenient with myself. Another photo sticks in my mind: a sixth grader, cheerful, chubby with a cowlick boinged above, snaggle-toothed smile, and a few zits on my dairy-fed face, and don't forget the Hang Ten shirt. Seeing only the defects and none of the wholesome confidence my school picture radiated, my 11-year-old self hid the school photo under a bedroom rug, where dirt and sand slowly ground into it, defacing it. There was no love there.

Yet another photo from time's album: me in first grade, in glorious black and white, clip-on bow tie. I'm as skinny as can be—angular face, tuberculosis-thin. I had no awareness of fat or thin. Just a kid, careless of such things. All that was about to change (let's have a few ominous chords from Beethoven's fifth).

My family had visited my aunt and uncle in Southern California. My aunt was proud of maintaining a svelte, youthful appearance. Every day it took her an hour to "put her face on," and she kept trim. My mom was, well, the mom, prone to fluctuations of the flesh, and other priorities enabled her to tolerate a less-than-perfect body. They were polar opposites: my aunt's Laurel to Mom's Hardy. Get my mom and aunt together and the topic of weight always received inordinate attention. They would talk about themselves losing or gaining, or the bodily vicissitudes of this or that movie star or family member.

Together they commented, "Grady is starting to have a paunch." Before that, I had innocently observed a little contour of flesh developing and it seemed kind of cute, something to be proud of. Now, with the strident commentaries, it became the paunch from the Black Lagoon.

Scales of Doom

My cousin echoed it, and later back at home a babysitter verified it. Astringent words like diet and exercise came into my lexicon. It was a pivotal moment, during that visit to Taft, the poor man's Bakersfield, when I went from being unselfconsciously at one with my body to being conflicted, a vessel that harbored spite for that growing pillow of flesh between my belly button and abdomen.

No sooner had we got home from the trip to Taft, I stepped on the rusty puke-green bathroom scales and weighed myself. Then I planted my feet on this tiny square platform spray-painted in gold, mounted on a ball-bearing swivel base. A silhouetted narrow-waisted female figure was stenciled on the platform, ringed by stars, and here, upon the Trim Twist, you could shimmy and pretzel yourself back and forth, swivel those hips and shed the pounds.

After ten minutes of mind-numbing gymnastic monotony, a mild sweat had broken out on my forehead. I got off the Trim Twist and headed straight to the bathroom scales. I had already lost maybe a gram of weight. At this rate, I concluded it would take approximately 77 years of shimmying on the Trim Twist to attain slimness.

From Taft to Watsonville is a journey of four hours in automobile, yet for me it had been a bullet train from carefree to morose. By listening to those family voices, I relinquished my personal power to the scales, and my self-regard took an enormous hit; I was wedded to an exasperating attachment to instant results and a festering discontent directed at me, *as I am*, the baseline for okayness.

Part of my childhood happiness had now been robbed by a needle that lined up against a wheel of ascending numbers. And my full future happiness was held hostage by those numbers. Sensing the hopelessness, I said the heck with diets and exercise. I was seven years old.

All the Candy

As a grade-schooler I blossomed into an all-American gourmand, gorging on cheeseburgers, fries, chocolate shakes, banana splits, and tons of candy. Dad had a drug store where my sister, our friends, and I had our pick of the bars and chocolate: U-no bars, Almond Roca, Milk Duds, Boston Baked Beans, Baby Ruth, Peanut Butter Cups and Hershey's. Every time we went to Dad's drug store it was a child's dream come true of being set loose in a candy store.

In grade school, I was a dismal failure at all sports, but one: all-you-can-eat buffets. It was considered success to load the plate and shovel it down; a real source of pride. I was often accused of having "eyes bigger than my stomach," but never of failing to clean the plate.

True, there abounded great periods of oblivious, happy childhood on the Central California coast. The fat thing became this sore spot that sporadically inflamed, triggered by impending visits from my aunt, uncle and cousin. Panic set in. There'd be the inevitable, "You've put on more weight," or my cousin's rendition of *fatty fatty two by four*. He knew, having a child's unerring instinct for inflicting cruelty, it would get my goat.

Crueler still were the airwaves that could turn something fun into unadulterated lousiness without warning. It still hurts to re-member a grueling scene in *To Sir With Love,* where a bullying gym teacher makes the spastic fat boy jump over the vaulting horse. My whole extended family was watching the movie on TV and this triggered a spate of comments about my weight and lack of athletic ability.

To balance things out, now and again would come the beneficent bolt from the blue: "You've slimmed down." The remark would bring a windfall surge of well-being. But since I didn't know what I had done to cause this, or rather, had done nothing consciously to lose weight—this undeserved good feeling was transitory and due to something entirely out of my control. Like the weather.

Brainwashed

In point of fact, I was never obese, but overweight. Hefty, chubby, or stocky. (That's a good one. Stocky is like calling somebody fat without the stigma.) For me, the physical reality was unimportant; what was devastating was an aching *awareness* of being over-weight, the identity more than the reality. I had been brain-washed and bought into all those wanton voices describing me as fat. In short, I had learned to be un-okay with myself and was easy prey to dermatologists and orthodontists.

By the fourth grade, the family doctor put me on thyroid tablets— another bit of medical sorcery. Blaming excess weight on the sluggish function of a gland in my neck and trying to induce weight loss with a bitter powdery tiny white tablet that I couldn't ever swallow, not even when ensconced in a slice of bread, served to reinforce the fact that my weight was A PROBLEM and that it was now related to physiological factors beyond my control. Like a police copter hovering over the hood, the weight was always on my to-do list, and I never got around to dealing with it. Those extra pounds stood between me and contentment. They booby-trapped my childhood pleasures. A good time could turn instantly into a rotten time whenever somebody opened their mouth and said the wrong thing.

I remember sitting down at an all-you-can-eat smorgasbord in Bakersfield, plate fully loaded, anticipating with delight fried chicken and hot buttered biscuits and spaghetti and salad loaded with croutons and chunky blue cheese, a tall cup of ice-packed fountain Coca-Cola, and my sparrow-thin aunt commented, gazing at me, "Some people really enjoy eating."

In my ears, at a moment when I was just raising my first forkful of food to my watering mouth, it became a withering indictment of one of life's pleasures. It became an indictment of this very moment: like I was supposed to not look like I was enjoying this.

Crash Diet

When I was 15 and weighed over 230 pounds, I returned to my small hometown, fresh from my first extended tour of L.A., Hollywood and Beverly Hills. Driven by a desire to be attractive and to find out about this thing called sex, I decided to make a change. So I accepted all the punishing clichés involved in the popular conception of diet. I drastically reduced my food portions and dramatically increased physical activity. I had one whole summer to bicycle and develop a serious bathroom scale fetish—the rusting puke-green device would be consulted on every conceivable occasion—after defecating, after feasting, in the morning, noon and night. Both naked and clothed.

As the numbers on the scale crept downward, I started hearing utterances like "svelte" and "slender" and "you're losing your baby fat." This last remark from the constituency of people who attributed the physical change to nature and not a regimen of 13-miles cycling, once or twice a day. When I got back to high school in September—I was a rock star. My world changed, doors opened. I had slayed the dragon.

Nevertheless, I hadn't modified habits. Snacking and exercising right after having lunch and increasing the amount of exercise in proportion to how much I had eaten—all these constituted a punishment cycle. For example, after wolfing down a Polynesian TV dinner and eating half a loaf of bread, wiping up the sweet sauce from the dinner with each buttered slice, I would do 100 sit-ups. Even after all the cycling and weight loss, periodic chain-eating still persisted: one Frito after another, one cookie after another. I still loved to guzzle a quart of milk.

I did, however, heed my aunt's advice, "Whenever you see the scales creeping up, cut back right away."

Learning to Love

Although amazingly, I managed to maintain a steady weight of around 180-190 pounds while perpetuating a cycle of sin, punishment, and self-imposed starvation, I was still far from loving and accepting myself.

It took me twenty years—a fifth of a century—to reach that state of okayness. When, free of anxiety about perceived fat, I started to exercise in the morning, to eat fresh, and commenced the process that would enable me to lose sixty pounds and six pants sizes in one year.

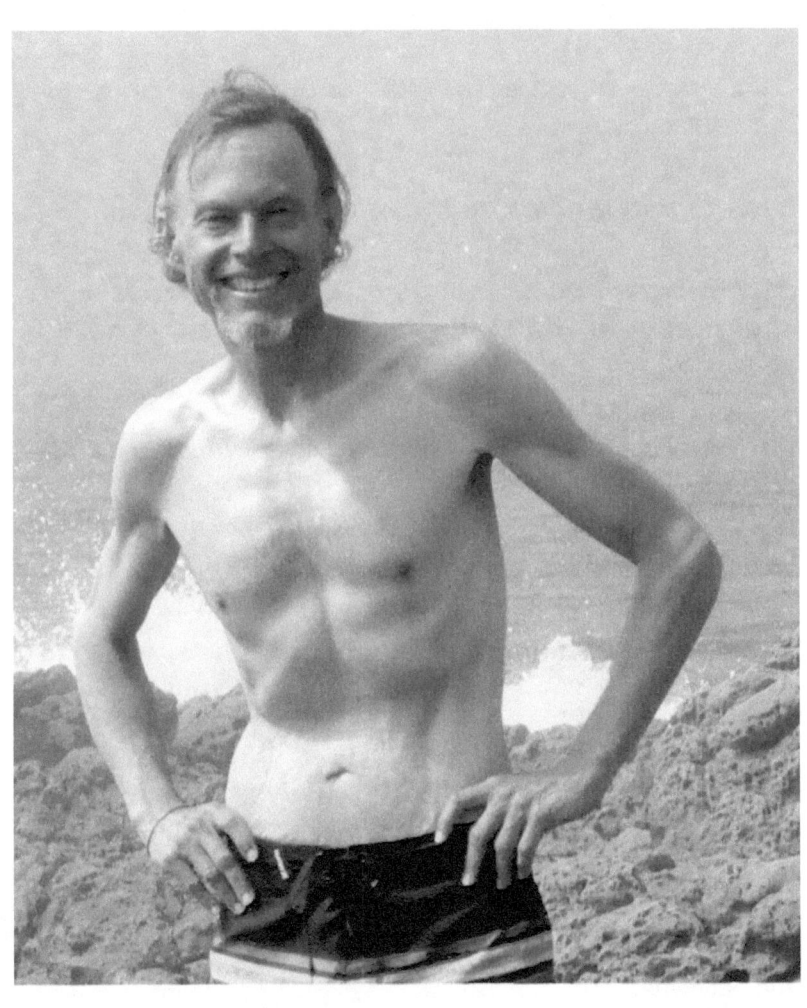

Today, livin' the life of Grady. . .

May this book help you progress and reach the knowledge:

Each moment is a clean slate.

Each moment gives us the opportunity to forgive ourselves.

Each moment gives us the opportunity to laugh.

Each moment gives the opportunity to exercise choice in both what goes in our mouth and what comes out of our mouth.

And, more importantly, what comes out of our minds.

Others' words we can take or leave.

What we're thinking and telling ourselves, we take to heart.

So, be careful about what you tell yourself. Be vigilant. And most of all, be kind.

I'm talking about our actions and our words. Actions: like choosing nuts over sweets. Words: carefully watch what you are saying and believing.

When it comes to diet and nutrition, silence is often preferable. There are many times when I'd counsel you to please be quiet about it. We've got a nation full of people who classify themselves as obese and who constantly chatter about the diet they can't stick to and how many calories this or that.

I tell you: if you talk about food, freely praise its qualities, its deliciousness, its scrumptiousness. Don't excuse it or vilify it. Bless it, be thankful. Love and celebrate each step of your personal evolution—even the missteps. Love yourself. Love and accept your body. Now. In fact, tattoo these words on your soul:

EVERY BODY

IS PERFECT

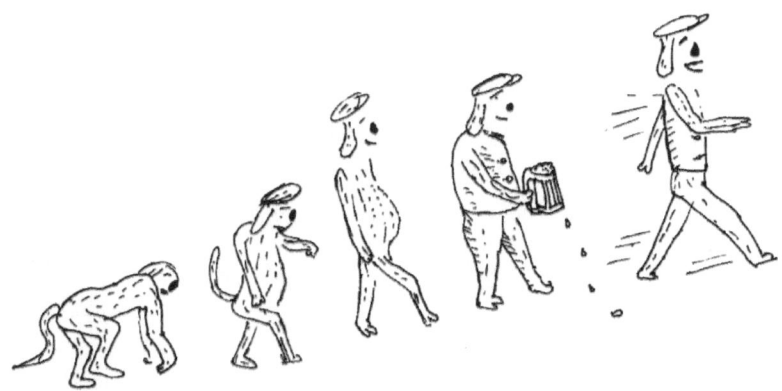

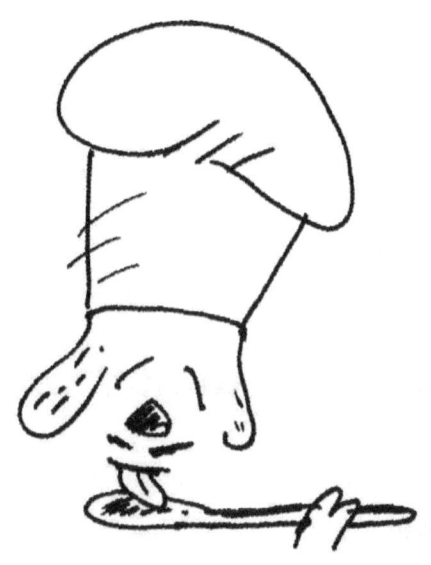

10. THE GRADY KOOKBOOK

EAT THE GRADY WAY

START WITH A PLATE, a nice big dinner plate. Use that for your salads. And when it comes to the "main" course (i.e. the meat), more than half of the plate can be occupied by the vegetable portion. Get used to using a big plate to form the measure for your fruits and veggies. It's a physical counterpart to the dietary changes you're making to put good things into your body.

From now on, as you adopt a new way of eating and living, you will be rebels and in direct opposition to the culinary status quo. Indeed, you will be asserting your independence while embedded within a world that talks the health talk and the thinness talk 'til it's blue in the face while consistently failing to walk the talk. That takes guts.

When it comes to eating out, learn to forego the mashed potato and rice for a double veggie portion. Instead of hash browns at breakfast, ask for tomato slices.

When you get accustomed to the big plate and generous portion of fruits and vegetables, it's hard not to get miffed at restaurants that measure out miserly fruit and veggie portions. I'll admit I've caused scenes at a Thai restaurant on Melrose and, more recently, at a breakfast place I enjoy in Toluca Lake, where I decided to order the fruit plate instead of the cup. I received what you see below and ended up asking for more. (OK, I'd already eaten two grapes when I took the picture.)

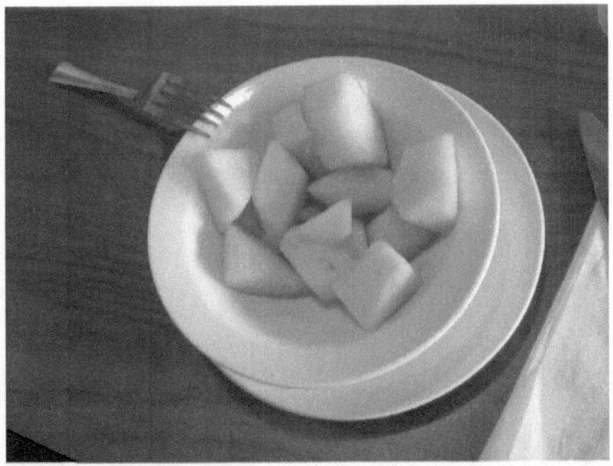

Without being rude or unkind, we have a duty to educate restaurants when it comes to proper fruit and veggie servings.

INTO THE KITCHEN

Your Best Friend: A Vegetable Steamer

Folks, it took me years to figure out what this device does and its purpose. It was a total mystery.

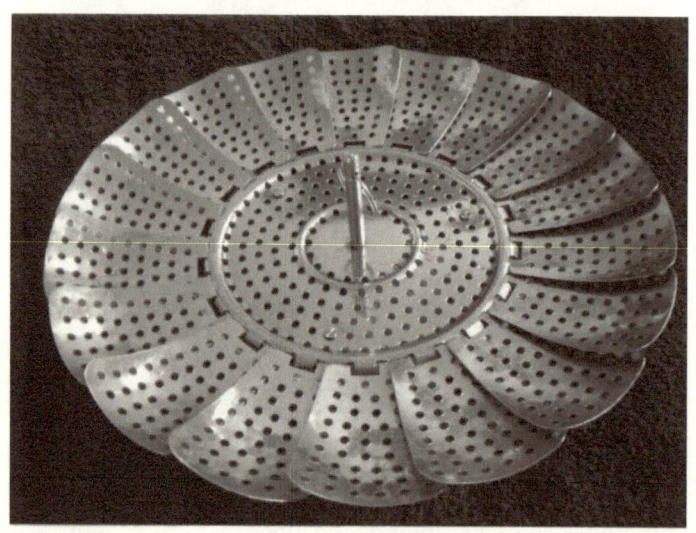

This goes in the bottom of a pot filled with half an inch of water, give or take. The steam rises through the holes and cooks the vegetables. Put it on a stove and use this to steam all the vegetables you like, even apples and yams. 10 to 20 minutes should do it, depending on taste. Do you like veggies soft and mushy or *al dente*—firm to the bite? Then give it five minutes.

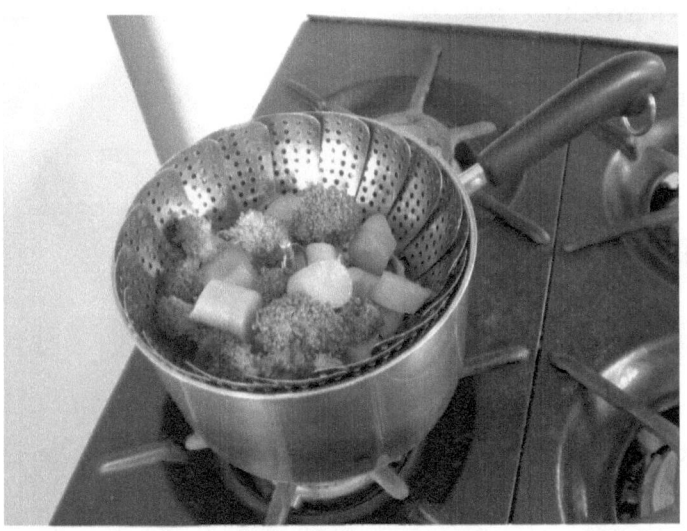

Get yourself a steamer and go wild in the kitchen, creating your own recipes. Determine how well done you like your veggies. Small slices cook faster. Larger pieces are said to have better flavor.

MEASUREMENTS

My preferred measurement for a single person's serving is a half cup of beans, oatmeal, rice, etc. It seems like a small measure, before cooking, but it magically turns out to be a lot. You might even have leftovers.

Even if you think you don't have a special cup for measuring, you do. Look at it this way: A cup is 8 ounces—the size of a regular small coffee or drink cup. So if you have a small disposable coffee or drink cup, you already have a measuring cup.

Spoons come in two sizes. The small one is a teaspoon. The large is a soup spoon, which kitchen folk call a tablespoon. For those uncouth people like myself who may lack both kinds of spoon, here are my easy equivalents: a beer cap – you know, the metal, serrated kind.

1 beer cap = 1/2 teaspoon

3 beer caps = one tablespoon

Some of my recipes mention the measurement a *handful*. Be assured, whatever your handful is, it's the right one.

SALADS

Growing up a California kid, salads are a staple before many meals. So much so, I almost forgot to include them. My favorite ingredients: tomatoes, celery, spinach, carrots, broccoli, onions, avocadoes and beets.

Grady Salad

Sliced beets
Garbanzo beans

Who says you need greens to make a salad? This is my answer. Mix half a can of garbanzo beans with half a can of beets.

Classic Salad

Lettuce or spinach
Chopped tomatoes
Chopped carrots
Chopped celery

Place a handful of each ingredient in a bowl. Cool way to chop celery: keep all the stalks together and chop from the top till you have a handful to add to your salad.

Dressing: As you like. My faves are: olive oil + a spoonful of mayo; soy and drops squeezed from a fresh lemon; olive oil + ketchup.

MEAT DISHES

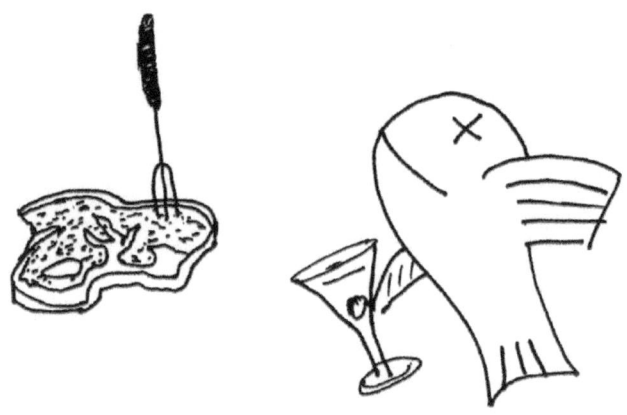

When people see my slender body, they falsely assume that I'm a strict vegetarian. Nothing could be further from the truth. Let me share some of my favorite carnivorous recipes with you.

Presto Chicken

Popeyes Chicken & Biscuits: **www.popeyes.com**

They've got spicy and mild fried chicken, slaw and green bean sides. Love the red beans. (You'd do well to forget the biscuits.)

Fast Burgers

Going to one of the burger chains is OK. Here's what you do. Most of them now offer a generic garden salad. Order the salad and a burger. To drink: ask for the complementary water for before or after your meal.

When the burger comes, discard the buns and put them in the garbage. Or discard one bun, if you so prefer. The thing is to exercise CHOICE. Always weave your own CHOICES into your eating.

Place the burger patty atop the salad. And one last thing: Enjoy!

One Southern California burger chain, In-N-Out Burger, serves 'protein' burgers. Instead of a bun, crisp iceberg lettuce wraps an all-beef patty, garnished with tomato and fresh onion slices. This awesomely fresh tasting burger goes perfectly with the Grady

Diet. So look for something similar where you live. And if you can't find it, request that it be added to the menu.

Veggie Tuna Delight

Let's hear it for tuna fish. It comes in handy single-serving cans, ideal for people on the run. The ingredients for the Veggie Tuna Delight are:

One can of tuna
One handful chopped celery
One handful chopped tomato
One half of an avocado, sliced
One handful diced onions
One sliced fresh jalepeño

Empty the contents of the tuna can into a bowl and combine all the other ingredients. And you've got a great main dish.

MORE MAINS

A Full Meal – Slaw and Soup

An easy-to-prepare full meal is slaw and soup. This classic combo is especially nice on a cold cloudy day. (Yes, we do have cold cloudy days even in sunny Southern California.)

Less than 1-Hour Split Pea Soup

1/2 cup of split peas

Four cups of water

A handful of chopped onion

A handful of sliced carrot

1/2 teaspoon (i.e. one beercap) of salt

The quick and easy way to make slaw and soup is make the slaw yourself and buy a can of split-pea soup at the market.

OR

You'll want to prepare the soup first, which will require, all told, about an hour of thinking ahead. Put the four cups of water in an open pot, add the half cup of dried split peas. Bring to a boil. (Leave the lid off for now. Split pea soup has an uncanny knack for boiling over. The instant your back is turned, there's suddenly a mess on your stove. A cleaning/cooking tip: When a mess occurs, immediately switch to a new burner, so the previous mess doesn't bake onto the burner.)

As soon as the water and split peas boil, reduce the heat to lowest simmer and put the lid on the pot. Let soup simmer for 30 minutes.

After the 30-minute low simmer, take the lid off and leave it off. Turn the stove to high and boil for twenty minutes. Stir occasionally, especially as the water steams away, so the peas won't burn to the bottom of your pot. Add the sliced carrot and onions toward the end of the cooking time if you like your cooked veggies crisper. After the final 20-minute high boil, you will have nice and creamy pea soup, ready to serve with the slaw.

Slaw

One cabbage (purple or white)
One carrot
One tablespoon of vinegar
One tablespoon of mayonnaise
Pepper

To prepare slaw, finely chop enough cabbage to fill a bowl, starting from the top of the cabbage head. (There'll be plenty of cabbage left for another day.) Add a tablespoon of vinegar and one tablespoon of mayonnaise. (A good mayo alternative is avocado mashed and mixed into the cabbage slaw.) Add a handful of diced bits of carrot for color and flavor. Then stir.

Pepper to your liking, and stir. Serve and eat.

As I am a rare combination of slob and efficiency expert, I like the fact that you can eat the slaw first, and then use the same bowl to serve the soup, thus eliminating the need to wash more dishes.

One-Hour Black Beans

Black beans are loaded with anthocyanins, antioxidants that have been shown to improve brain function. A 1/2-cup serving provides 8 grams of protein and 7.5 grams of fiber. It's also low in calories and free of saturated fat. *Blablabla*.

Let's start cooking. Gather your ingredients:

1/2 cup of black beans
Four cups of water
One garlic clove (chopped)
A handful of chopped onion
Salt (a beer cap, optional)

Bring the water and beans to a boil. Maintain a steady boil on medium heat for 20 minutes. KEEP THE LID OFF so it doesn't boil over.

Turn down the heat to low simmer. Place the lid on the pot and let it simmer for 40 minutes. Add the garlic and chopped onion when you begin to simmer the beans. This recipe makes beans the way I like them: tender and watery. Serve and eat.

Old-Fashioned Beans

1/2 a cup of beans
Water
Salt (your call)

Choose from pinto beans, kidney beans, fava beans or black beans. Soak the beans overnight. Put the beans in a pot and fill with water to three fingers above the beans.

Bring the pot to a boil and place a tilted lid on top. Keep the pot boiling on medium heat for an hour and a half, stirring the pot occasionally. Feel free to sample the beans to see if they are reaching the desired softness.

As the water steams away, keep adding new water as the beans boil. (An old trick is to keep a side pan of water heated, so you can add already hot water and not diminish the boil.)

Surprise Soup

A selection of all the veggies in your fridge
Salt and pepper (your call)
A bay leaf (highly recommended)
Four cups of water

This recipe is based on the steadfast belief that there's always something in the fridge or cupboard. If you think you need to go to the store, you're wrong. Look around and you'll be surprised by what you've already got.

Whatever you have in your vegetable compartment, take it out. Fill a pot with water, and add chopped veggies. Use as many parts of the vegetables as you can. For instance, if you have broccoli, chop the stem as well and add it to the pot. Add water and bring to a boil, putting on a tilted lid and lowering the heat to a simmer after a boil is first attained.

Let the soup simmer for 20 to 40 minutes, depending on how soft you like your vegetables. Celery is great. The leaves can be left on to add an extra zing of seasoning.

Tacos à la Grady

If there is a versatile veggie, it's cabbage; great for slaw and as an alternative tortilla. Cut the leaf at the stem, right near the base. Peel off a whole broad, curved cabbage leaf ideal for making a taco. It can be filled with beans or meat. I really like fried kosher ground beef or turkey in the cabbage wrap.

I'm sure cabbage is good for something health-wise, but why bore you with the details. From a culinary engineering standpoint, cabbage leaves are good for making tacos. What more do you need to know?

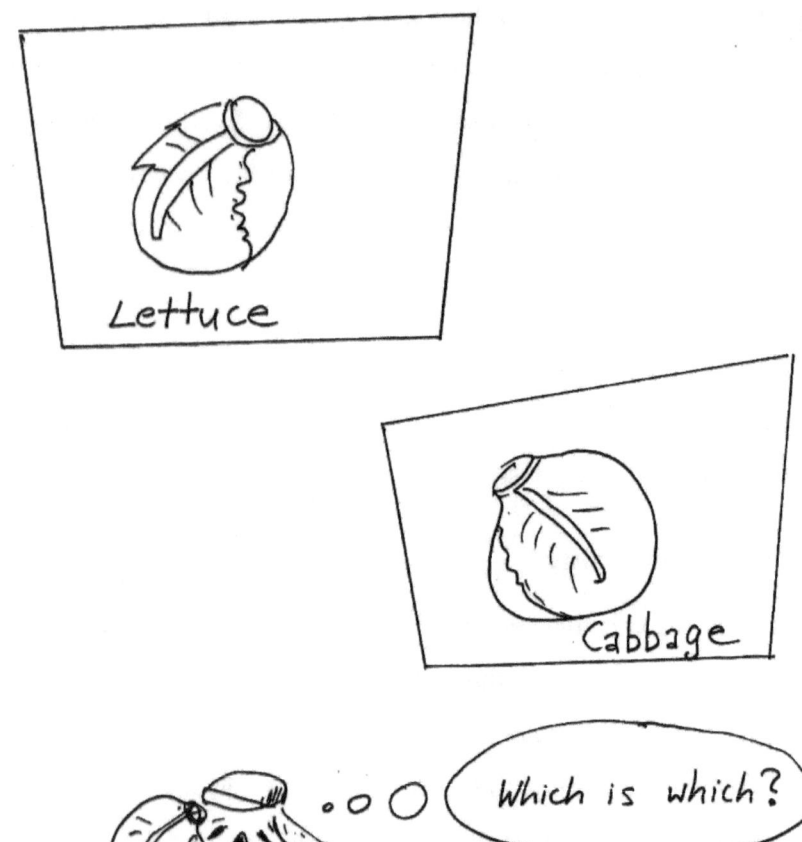

GOODIES

Sunmaid Scrabble

One cup of raw husked sunflower seeds.
1/2 cup of raisins.

Mix the two ingredients in a bowl and you have dessert. The fact is, if you like salted sunflower seeds, they make a great combo with the sweet raisins.

Monkey Mix

One cup of raw husked sunflower seeds.
One cup of banana chips.

This is a tasty alternative to the sunflower-raisin treat. The calories would be few, but let me emphasize that I discourage calorie counting. It's assigning a number for disapproval; it's a guilt rating. Who needs that?

Just count the things you want to grow.

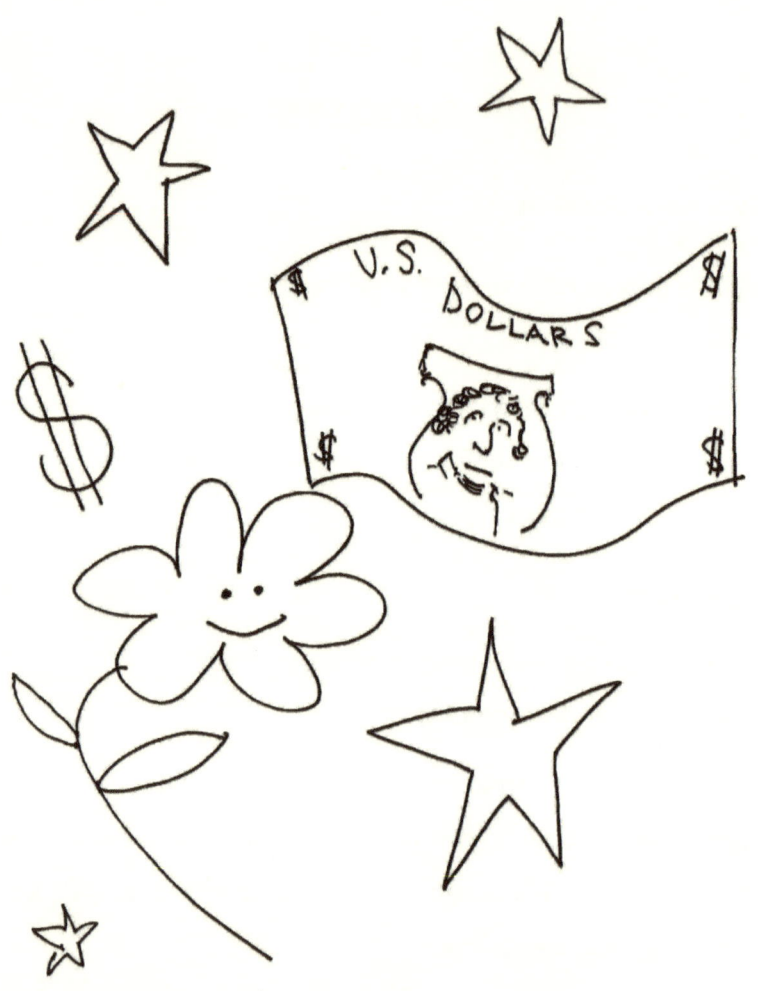

COUNT THE THINGS
YOU WANT TO GROW.

HOLIDAYS

Sooner or later the holidays will pounce on us, jingle bells pouring through our ears. The season unleashes its annual assault of leering glutens and poisonous confections, an unstoppable blitzkrieg of yummies designed to wear down the most obstinate health nut. Still, there *is* something you can do to preserve your waistline and your self-respect.

As a humorist and diet guru, let me remind you of one magical word:

CHOICE

You always have a choice. Always. You can pick the blueberries off the multiple-homicide divinity decadence torte and scuttle the rest in a cocktail napkin. You can take the top slice of bread off a sandwich, and eat it on one slice. When going to a party you can be charmingly eccentric and bring your own walnuts, packaged by nature, and your own nutcracker. Sure, you run the risk of being labeled a nut—no mean feat in Hollywood—but hey, you can always reply, "You're right—I am what I eat."

That said, even when you're eating well—fruits, veggies, and whole grains—the sweet stuff can be downright enticing during the holidays, which are a boot camp for exercising choice.

As a down-to-earth diet guru, I've enshrined within the three squares, snack time, your time for the chocolate chip cookie. And for the holidays, I've taken a few time-tested family favorites and given them a healthy twist.

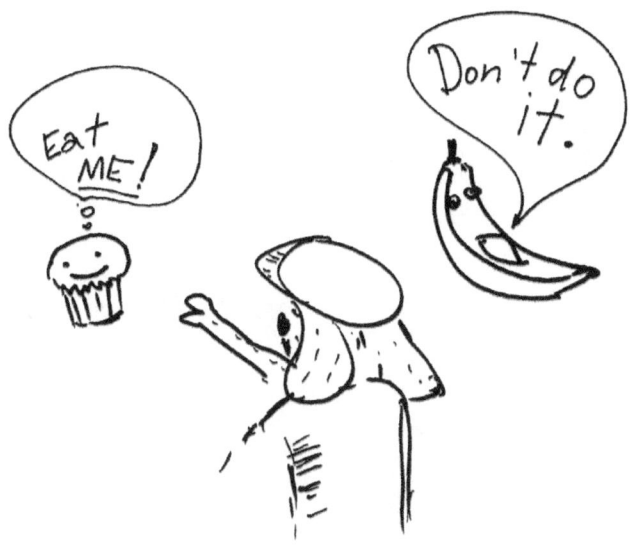

Scottish Whole-Wheat Shortbread

1/2 lb. butter

2 cups sifted whole wheat flour

1/2 cup powdered sugar

Place the four cups of flour into a bowl. Using very clean hands, work flour into the butter a little at a time—cream thoroughly. Add powdered sugar gradually—cream thoroughly. Handle *lightly*. (Too much handling causes the dough to become tough.) CHILL DOUGH for 30 minutes. Put on lightly floured board and spread to about ½" thick. Punch with fork prongs and cut into shapes.

Baking time depends some on your oven. The original recipe says to bake at 350° for five minutes, or 300° for 20 to 30 min.

Yogurt Pancakes

1/2 cup of whole-wheat flour

1/2 cup flax meal

One egg

One teaspoon (i.e. two beer caps) of baking powder or soda

One tablespoon (six beer caps) of olive oil

1/4 cup of yogurt

1/2 cup of water

Start with the flour and flax meal. Add the baking soda or powder. Add the egg and 1/4 cup of yogurt and save the 1/2 cup of water for last—so it washes out the yogurt in the measuring cup.

Stir all the while with a spoon. Keep stirring until the batter is smooth.

Heat a non-stick pan on a medium flame. (On a non-stick pan you theoretically don't need to use cooking oil. As the owner of semi-stick pans, I know better. So grease the pan with something.) Will make three large pancakes. Sweeten as you desire: real maple syrup, sugar free, honey, jelly, banana slices, or the toxic remnants of cookie dough from last year's school fundraiser. And I do like a pat of real dairy butter on top when the cakes are hot off the griddle.

Holiday Detox Smoothie

Three oranges
A handful of spinach

Juice the three oranges. Pour the juice of the three oranges into a blender. Add the handful of spinach. Mix in the blender until the juice turns a nice frothy green. (about 20 seconds at medium speed)

On a warm day enjoy on ice.

FURTHER READING

Viktor Frankl, *Man's Search for Meaning*

Louise L. Hay, *You Can Heal Your Life*

Megan Oaten and Ken Cheng, "Longitudinal gains in self-regulation from regular physical exercise," British Journal of Health Psychology (2006)
(**www.gpscbc.ca/system/files/Longitudinal%20gai ns%20in%20self-regulation.pdf**)

Michael O'Riordan, "Laughing Your Way to Lower Blood Pressure and Less Stress,"
(**www.theheart.org/article/865875.do**)

FURTHER LISTENING

Bernie S. Siegel, *Humor and Healing*

FURTHER VIEWING

"Laughter Yoga CNN report,"
(**www.youtube.com/watch?v=J5sSgdJIU5g&noredir ect=1**), an interview with Dr. Madan Kataria, founder of Laughter Yoga.

"The Science of Laughter" The Science of Laughter/ Mind/ Exploratorium TV
(**www.exploratorium.edu/tv/index.php?project=58 &program=543**) Interview with Dr. William Fry, Stanford University researcher who pioneered the study of laughter's health benefits.

"Telling Jokes in Auschwitz" – **the MY HERO Project (www.myhero.com/go/films/view.asp?film=jokesa uschwitz**) – *A man talks about his experiences in a concentration camp and how he chooses to look at life with humor instead of sorrow.*

Thank Yous:

Brad Wyman: You believed in the Grady Diet. Your vision took it from a humble pamphlet to a proud book, and you kindled the cartoonist in me. To **Matthew Barrett** for generous patience, superb editorial suggestions and your heroic role in rescuing the "lost" cartoons. **Ashley Rozatti**: your visual stamp on the manuscript and great contribution as cartoon muse remain. Thanks to **Michele R. Sadler** for exceptional proofreading; **Don Goodman**, for the awesome author's photo; **Jeffrey Davis** your talented lens and sage guidance. For soulful marketing genius, thank you **Paul David**. For wise observations, special thanks **Karen Valenti, Jonathan Sieger, Adrian Riskin, Carey Fosse.** Thanks **Yevgen Kaminsky** for the perfect interior art, using titles by visual wiz **Lex Munson**. Distinguished novelist **S.R. Mallery** gave illuminating suggestions that raised the whole quality of the print edition. Who but you can convey naked editorial truths and still amuse and encourage? I thank last but no less profusely **Vivek Rajan Vivek,** a wise man who lavishly shares the wisdom in his books and deeds. You made the dream of print real for me, and your eye-popping cover will continue to blaze this book's way to the hearts of many readers.

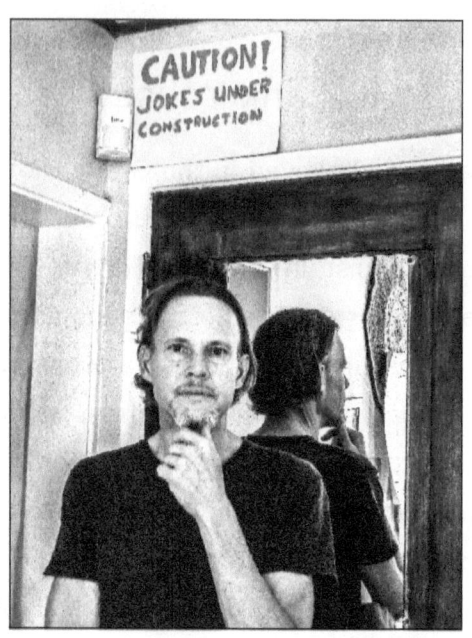

Photo by Don Goodman

ABOUT THE AUTHOR

Hollywood Humorist Grady Miller has been compared to T.C. Boyle, Joel Stein, and Voltaire. He attended Columbia University, which he fled before graduating. He came to Los Angeles to study filmmaking, but discovered literature instead, in T.C. Boyle's fiction writing workshop at USC. In addition to *Lighten Up Now*, Grady Miller has written a thriller, *The Hostages of Veracruz* (available on Amazon), as well as the popular humor collection, *Late Bloomer*, and its follow-up, the forthcoming *Later Bloomer*. His humor column, *Miller Time,* appears weekly in The Canyon News.

(**www.canyon-news.com**)